COLLOIDAL MINERALS AND TRACE ELEMENTS

COLLOIDAL MINERALS AND TRACE ELEMENTS

How to Restore the Body's Natural Vitality

MARIE-FRANCE MULLER, M.D., N.D., Ph.D.

Translated by Jon Graham

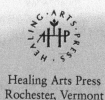

Healing Arts Press
Rochester, Vermont

Healing Arts Press
One Park Street
Rochester, Vermont 05767
www.InnerTraditions.com

Healing Arts Press is a division of Inner Traditions International

Originally published in French under the title *Minéraux et oligo-éléments collóidaux source de santé vitalité et jouvence* by Éditions Jouvence, S.A., Chemin du Guillon 20, Case 143 CH-1233 Bernex, Switzerland, www.editions-jouvence.com, info@editions-jouvence.com
First U.S. edition published in 2005 by Healing Arts Press

Note to the reader: This book is intended as an informational guide. The remedies, approaches, and techniques described herein are meant to supplement, and not to be a substitute for, professional medical care or treatment. They should not be used to treat a serious ailment without prior consultation with a qualified health care professional.

LIBRARY OF CONGRESS CATALOGING-IN-PUBLICATION DATA

Muller, Marie-France.
[Mineraux et oligo-elements collóidaux. English]
Colloidal minerals and trace elements : how to restore the body's natural vitality / Marie-France Muller ; translated by Jon Graham.
p. cm.
Originally published in French under the title Mineraux et oligo-elements collóidaux.
Includes bibliographical references and index.
ISBN 978-1-59477-023-4 (pbk.)
1. Minerals in human nutrition. 2. Trace elements in the body. 3. Dietary supplements. 4. Colloids. I. Title.
QP533.M8413 2005
613.2'85—dc22
2004026769

Printed and bound in the United States

10   9   8   7   6

Text design and layout by Virginia Scott Bowman and Rachel Goldenberg
This book was typeset in Sabon with Brittanic, Delphin, and Avenir as display typefaces

CONTENTS

PART 3
Minerals: Building Blocks for Health

ACKNOWLEDGMENTS

I dedicate this book, the first of mine to be published in English, to my wonderful American family—to all of you who are directly descended or are related to the Mougin family of eastern France: Mougin, Brennan, Conlin, Gauthier, Jambora, Kelleher, Knapp, LeBlanc, Miler, Pastoreck, Rice, Tyrell, Curtis, Smyth, and all others.

I dedicate this to the remembrance of the fantastic journey of September 2004 that brought us all together and in particular to:

Eugene and Theresa Mougin, who are so close to my heart.

My cousins Dona Rice, Marcy Brennan, and Lynn Jambora, who are truly almost sisters to me, and to their children, Christine and Tom Smyth; Timothy and Kara Rice; Sadie, Meaghan and Kara Brennan; and Rick, Scott, and Brian Jambora.

Viviane Mougin Tyrell, whose sweet smile stands out in my memory, and to her large family, including Carol, Raymond, Thomas, Joan, Dorothy, Robert, Richard, Patricia, Marlene, Constance, Ronald, John, and Barbara.

Lenny Gauthier and her children, Laurie, John, and Chipper.

Jim and Roberta Gauthier (and the great times we shared together) and their children, Jimmy, Joel, and Julia.

The big-hearted Ed Miller and his family, including Bill, Bob, Edmund, John Miller, and Marilyn Curtis, and to all your children and grandchildren.

With the pass of a magic wand, you have enlarged my family to a whole new size and a whole new continent.

FOREWORD

Over the last 30 years, increasing numbers of Americans, particularly those with life-threatening illnesses, have begun to look for healthcare answers in complementary and alternative approaches. They are not turning their back on conventional medicine—it is, in fact, those who have had all the benefits of modern scientific medicine who have led the search—but they are very much aware of its limitations and side effects. They are exploring approaches that would complement this medicine—or in some cases, be alternatives to it.

FINAL REPORT OF THE WHITE HOUSE COMMISSION ON
COMPLEMENTARY AND ALTERNATIVE MEDICINE POLICY,
MARCH 2002

Demystifying the role of colloidal minerals, trace elements, and supplements by understanding their relationship to disease prevention and the maintenance and improvement of human health is a complex but essential task that needs to be undertaken in order to advance the science of integrative medicine.

All interested observers know that the database of medical knowledge has grown tremendously over the last two decades, with an increasing emphasis on understanding and diagnosing disease; an increasing awareness of the vast complexity of the regulatory mechanisms that govern cellular homeostasis, response, and function; and a greater reliance on the use of technology or extremely sophisticated medical interventions to manage and treat our patients. In the shadow of all these advances in traditional allopathic medicine lie the virtually untapped role of nutraceuticals and the increasingly popular interest in Complementary and Alternative Medicine (CAM).

According to the United States Food and Drug Administration (FDA), the definition of a dietary supplement is "any product taken by mouth that contains a so-called dietary ingredient and its label clearly states that it is a dietary supplement. The 'dietary ingredients' in dietary supplements may include vitamins, minerals, herbs, colloidal minerals, trace elements and amino acids as well as substances such as enzymes, organ tissues, metabolites, extracts or concentrates. Dietary supplements can be found in many forms such as pills, tablets, capsules, liquids or powders. They must be identified on the label as a dietary supplement." A good working definition of a nutraceutical is a dietary supplement to which pharmaceutical-grade clinical research is applied. In the United States and around the globe, nutraceuticals are usually acquired by patients independent of their physicians. These patients opt to "self-medicate" without necessarily having adequate product efficacy and safety data or even general information about the specifics of the compounds. This can be a prescription for disaster especially if the patient has multiple comorbidities and is already taking some type of prescription drug. An in-depth understanding of the safety and efficacy of these compounds can be achieved only through rigorous testing. Research into nutraceuticals is therefore absolutely essential.

The interest in nutraceuticals is one indication of the marked change in patients' perception of the medical establishment during the last fifteen years. People have become dissatisfied with the care provided by their physicians and the apparent restriction of physician services. In response to the strict control of managed care coupled with mixed results of treatment efficacy, the general public has started to use more CAM therapies, in particular herbal/nutritional supplements. A landmark study published in the *Journal of the American Medical Association* in 1998 by Dr. Eisenberg, director of the Center for Alternative Medicine Research and Education and assistant professor of medicine at Harvard examines trends in alternative medicine use in the United States between 1990 and 1997. It reported that the prevalence of

CAM use increased from 33 percent in 1990 to 42.1 percent in 1997. The total number of visits to CAM providers during this period increased from 427 million in 1990 to 629 million in 1997. Furthermore, multiple reports during the past five years confirm that the range of CAM usage is broadening and that currently 50–80 percent of the U.S. population has used some form of CAM therapy. Nearly three quarters of such patients use it in conjunction with traditional medical care; the remaining quarter seeks such treatments as a replacement for traditional care.

In response to the growing demands of consumers seeking alternative medicine, hospitals and academic medical centers are adding CAM services to improve patient satisfaction. Today, an estimated 20 percent of U.S. hospitals offer alternative therapies and nearly 100 academic medical centers have CAM clinics.

CAM therapies are usually self-prescribed with no communication occurring between the patient and his or her primary care physician. Integrative medicine, in contrast, incorporates CAM therapies under the guidance of an MD (medical doctor), DO (osteopath), or ND (naturopathic doctor) who has training in integrative therapies. It is a healing-oriented medicine that draws upon all therapeutic systems to form a comprehensive approach to the art and science of medicine under the supervision of one of these three practitioners.. Integrative medicine combines the benefits of both conventional medicine and CAM therapies, including the use of nutraceuticals, to benefit the patient's health and well-being.

But how does all this relate to this book, *Colloidal Minerals and Trace Elements?* Credible, accurate, evidence-based information on colloidal minerals and trace elements (nutraceuticals) is essential to facilitate a new era of modern medicine that includes healthier patients and a healthier relationship between practitioner and patient.

Medicine is dynamic and always changing. The ability to analyze, understand, and incorporate new information into healthcare strategies is essential for progress. As Oliver Wendell Holmes has said, "Greatness is not in where we stand . . . but in what direction we are moving."

Colloidal Minerals and Trace Elements by Marie-France Muller is an essential reference and practical guide for patients and physicians interested in the latest knowledge regarding these nutrients. It provides much-needed and valuable historical, anecdotal, and scientific information on how to incorporate these substances into our daily lives to restore the body's natural vitality.

JOSEPH V. PERGOLIZZI JR., M.D.,
ADJUNCT ASSISTANT PROFESSOR,
JOHNS HOPKINS UNIVERSITY SCHOOL OF MEDICINE;
EDITOR IN CHIEF, *CLINICAL RESEARCHER*

IN THE KINGDOM OF THE INFINITELY SMALL

No cellular functions can be produced correctly if the body isn't receiving all the minerals and trace elements the metabolism needs. . . . It so happens that all degenerative diseases originate, to one degree or another, in a severe mineral depletion of the body.

Dr. Robert LaFave,
U.S. Metabolic Research Center

Minerals (mineral salts) are necessary for life. They are essential in all life's functions. From the dawn of time, humans and animals alike have always eaten their minerals and trace elements, including the rare earths (in the form of clays), various salts, animal tissue (flesh and bones), and plants that are rich in colloidal minerals—minerals in that soluble suspended state necessary for plants and all living organisms to be able to absorb them from the soil. As it stands today, our arable land is sick and anemic from our misuse and can no longer provide us with everything we need.

The resulting depletion and imbalance of minerals in our bodies is the source of most of our current ailments. This is something that numerous researchers have asserted again and again for more than a century, although their efforts have far too often gone unheard. If we can right this deplorable state of affairs and restore to ourselves a lifestyle that is more in keeping with the one humanity has known for most of its long history, we may envision the possibility of all of us recovering the vitality we may have lost on the road of modern life, and living to a ripe old age while preserving both our faculties and the energy we need to enjoy them.

The premise of this book is that trace elements (the metalloids or metallic elements that represent only the smallest percentage of the constitutions of living organisms) and minerals, especially when absorbed in a natural, colloidal form, can allow us to make an extraordinary leap forward toward better health and well-being. It seems that the depletion of these essential elements is enough to disturb the working order of all the body's systems. But when the body's needs for them are met, it is rapidly able to return to a state of ideal functioning.

Of course, this level of our body's operation is one of life's smallest kingdoms. Here in this domain, it is not quantity that counts as much as a complete and balanced intake of all the minerals we need—as well as their quality and our ability to absorb them easily. *Oligotherapy* is that therapeutic method based on supplying the body with minerals or trace elements to achieve the balance necessary for normal cell function.

In this book, we will journey to the center of the earth that feeds the very cells of all the life it carries so that we can gain a better understanding of the mechanisms connecting us to our planet through the intermediary of the foods we eat, the water we drink, and the air we breathe. It is obvious that the threatened health of our planet cannot help but have serious repercussions on our own well-being. Thus we shall also explore why we can no longer envision ourselves as a species apart and how our physical, mental, and energetic balance depends on the symbiosis we create with all other living things.

We will take a long look at colloidal trace elements that exist in perfectly balanced proportions within natural sources, which allows the body to recognize them as the true foods it needs in order to maintain or recover a perfect energetic balance. Though we all too often forget, our body is like an electrical system that requires all its components to perform well. If they don't, however, a breakdown or even a permanent outage is definitely in the cards.

I invite the reader to join me in this exploration of one of the world's smallest kingdoms: that of the minerals, the essential catalysts for sound body function.

PART I

Minerals and Trace Elements: Why Our Diet is Lacking These Important Nutrients

I

A BRIEF HISTORY

STONES THAT HEAL

The importance of minerals to the body's functioning is not a new concept. In fact, the use of stones and minerals for healing purposes reaches far back in time.

Ancient peoples were not satisfied to wear precious stones simply for the purpose of adornment, nor did they use them only as religious symbols. Such stones were also employed to maintain health and heal illnesses: They would be placed on whatever area of the body required healing or, if internal use was called for, would be administered in the form of a powder to be taken orally (please note that this method of treatment is not advised and can be dangerous) or in the form of a drink in which a specific stone had been soaked for a time. Another method involved simply giving patients water from a vessel that had been made from the appropriate stone for their condition.

Records of stones with medicinal properties can be found in the Assyrian, Chaldean, Egyptian, Indian, and Chinese pharmacopoeias. In the last we can cite, among other stones and clays, the use of alum for treating the lung and large intestine meridians, orpiment (arsenic sulfide) for treating the liver meridian, and red clay used in the treatment of dysentery and diarrhea.

In 6000 B.C.E., Chaldean priests chose which metal tablets to give to those suffering from illness based primarily on the planetary correspondences of the metal and the patients' affected organs.

A CEASELESS FERMENT OF ENERGY

In his book *Médecines ésoteriques, médecines de demain* (Paris: Éditions Denoël, 1976) Doctor Jacques Michaud tells us of a curious experiment:

Some years ago a jeweler, who was also an enthusiast of home movies, filmed what was taking place inside precious stones (diamonds) and thereby revealed to some stupefied scientists the ceaseless ferment of energy that animated these so-called inert masses. The esoteric sciences, however, did not have to wait for this particular revelation to grasp the enormous potentialities that minerals hold within.

Thirty-six hundred years ago, Melampus of Argos restored the Argosean king Iphiclus's lost virility by having him drink a cup of wine in which a piece of iron had been steeped—an early example of oligotherapy, but there are countless others like it in the records of all ancient civilizations.

The same was true in the Middle Ages, when the doctrine of signatures (analogies) was used to determine which mineral or precious stones were called for by a patient's condition. For example, obsidian was indicated for skeletal disorders, while ruby and gold—the preeminent solar metal—were indicated for the heart. According to Marbodius (an eleventh-century bishop), jasper was reputed to aid pregnant women, agate restored vigor to the man who wore it, emerald soothed passions and disorders affecting the liver and bile ducts, ruby made its wearer joyful, amethyst was beneficial to the brain (especially after heavy drinking!), and chalcedony could cure certain forms of delirium. These distinctions can give us a whole new perspective on the choice of stones we like to wear.

PARACELSUS AND HERMETIC MEDICINE

While the avowed purpose of alchemy is the transmutation of lead into gold, it has also given birth to a variety of mineral elixirs whose healing properties have been highly valued both in the past and in the present.

Paracelsus made great use of minerals, and not only in his alchemical operations. Starting in 1528, he created the foundations for a mineral-based medicine derived from alchemical principles. To a certain extent he was the father of metallotherapy. Few may know that it was he who named zinc or that even at this early date he was prescribing iron for the treatment of anemia and lead for the dressing of wounds. The basis of this medicine is the law of correspondences, wherein each sign of the zodiac and each planet corresponds to an organ of the body or it's function, as well as to one of the major metals:

PARACELSUS'S METAL–PLANET–BODY CORRESPONDENCES

METAL	PLANET	PART OF THE BODY
Gold	Sun	heart, spleen
Silver	Moon	esophagus, uterus, ovaries, lymphatic system, sympathetic nervous system
Iron	Mars	blood, hemoglobin, genital organs, left cerebral hemisphere, muscles, rectum
Copper	Venus	throat, kidney, thymus, venous blood circulation
Mercury	Mercury	bronchus, lungs, thyroid, tongue, cerebro-spinal system, sensitive nerves, right cerebral hemisphere, ears, eyes, breathing
Tin	Jupiter	liver, adrenal glands, arterial blood circulation
Lead	Saturn	gall bladder, teeth, joints, bones, skin, ligaments, sigmoid, pneumogastric nerve

Accordingly, in the case of cardiovascular problems, a preparation with a gold base was advised because of the correspondence between the heart and the sun. In this case, in the very words of Paracelsus, we must know how "to make the fixed volatile and then fix this volatile element in a preparation that can be *assimilated*." Even at this early date we find emphasis placed on this essential aspect of any mineral therapy—that is, the body's ability to assimilate or absorb the mineral. Paracelsus's spagyric* medicine, with its base of mineral and plant elixirs, was often credited for making miracles.

JUSTUS LIEBIG: A FORERUNNER

Turning now to a more "scientific" realm, it has been more than a century and a half since Justus Liebig traced the first glimmerings of the importance of minerals for health. Toward the middle of the nineteenth century, this savant who specialized in the study of plants had already tried to draw the attention of agriculturalists to the importance of alkaline elements, alkaline soils, and the phosphates necessary to plant growth. As he wrote: "These mineral principles are indispensable to the plant organism's ability to assimilate the nutritive substances with which the atmosphere provides it."[1]

Of course we now know that it is not only from the atmosphere that plants procure the nutritional substances they need, but also from the soil. This does not change the fact that Liebig put his finger on a basic notion that continues to fuel research.

THE WORK OF JACOB MOLESCHOTT

Some twenty years later another scholar, Jacob Moleschott, pursued Liebig's ideas even further in his book *The Circulation of Life:*

> The construction and vital capacity of organs are conditioned by the presence in necessary quantities of inorganic substances that are indispensable for their formation. This certitude allows me to assert without

---

*The term *spagyric* originates from the Greek *span* (to draw or pull, to separate) and *ageirein* (to bring together, collect, or unify). *Spagyrism* refers to a manufacturing process during which raw source materials obtained from mineral, plant, or animal sources are first separated and later reunited. The processes of cleansing and purification enable a form of medicine more effective than that possible on the basis of the original source materials.

Swiss-born alchemist and physician Phillippus Aureolus Theophrastus Bombast von Hohenheim (1493–1541), known in the modern day as Paracelsus, is associated with spagyric therapy.

pride or false modesty that the recently revealed importance of the relationship that exists between these mineral substances and the various parts of the body opens new horizons to the fields of both agriculture and medicine. It is indisputable, in the presence of the combined facts, that the mineral substances which remain in the ash following calcination play an essential role in the constitution—thus in the structure—of both the tissue and the substances that calcinations makes volatile.[2]

DOCTOR SCHÜSSLER'S BIOCHEMICAL SALTS

Born in 1821 in the Great Duchy of Oldenburg, Guillaume-Henri Schüssler became an initiate of homeopathy after having studied medicine in all the great capitals of Europe. Interested in the works of Liebig and Moleschott, in 1872 he began prescribing the mineral salts that researchers had shown took part in the composition of blood and tissue. In 1873 he published the first results of his new therapeutic method in his book *Abrégé de thérapeutique biochimique* (Abbreviated Biochemical Therapy).

Biochemistry is the study of the nature of vital conditions—those conditions necessary for life. Dr. Schüssler appropriately gave his name to his therapeutic method because its remedies were specifically and uniquely those mineral salts he identified whose presence in definite proportions is acknowledged as crucial to the formation and proper functioning of tissue. As he states in his book:

> Tissues are sick because the cells of which they are made no longer contain in the requisite proportions the mineral substances t hat are a factor in their constitution . . . Through the gradual intake of *weak doses* of these substances, the cells will be enabled to rebuild their structure and recover their vitality.[3]

Our cellular environment is composed of water that contains a number of dissolved substances of considerable biological importance. Some of the mineral substances that can be found there in the form of ions are charged positively, such as the cations (sodium, potassium, calcium, magnesium, for example), while others are charged negatively, such as the anions (chloride, sulfur, for example). Either a hyper- or a hypoconcentration of these constituent elements of the cell can prove disastrous. It is the consistency of these elements that determines good intercellular balance, and thus good health. Once a mineral imbalance occurs, the proper proportions between mineral elements and organic elements can no longer be maintained, which generally impedes optimum cellular function and leads to an excess of organic elements.

According to Schüssler's ideas, illness is created or accompanied by a deficiency in the quantity of cellular salts in living tissue and the resultant disorder in the molecular movement of these salts. Balance can be restored to these elements, order can be restored to these functions, and healing can thus be aided by administering these mineral salts in small amounts. As Schüssler understood it, if the mineral balance is disrupted,

> . . . the battle is definitively translated by a more or less significant loss
> of the cell's mineral elements. The ensuing pathological deterioration
> will be in direct proportion with the difficulties or possibilities the cell
> has in finding the means to remedy this situation more or less quickly
> within the intercellular environment.[4]

Known throughout the world as Dr. Schüssler's Tissue Salts or Tissulary Remedies and supposed to treat all human pathological conditions, these biochemical salts are offered in the form of powders or tablets (in packs of twelve) and include:

- Calcarea Phosphorica
- Calcarea Sulfurica
- Calcarea Fluorica
- Ferrum Phosphoricum
- Kali Muriaticum
- Kali Phosphoricum
- Kali Sulfuricum
- Magnesia Phosphorica
- Natrum Muriaticum
- Natrum Phosphoricum
- Natrum Sulfuricum
- Silicea

These tissue salts are in fact triturations of base minerals as found in nature, obtained through the homeopathic method—added to lactose and diluted to a potency of 6X (6 figures after the decimal point). Although his method is closely similar to that of Doctor Schüssler, he stated that his therapy was completely different from homeopathy:

> The disorders that occur in the metabolism of the mineral molecules
> of the human body are corrected in my method through the direct
> physical intake of the elements that are homogenous to the body,

whereas homeopathy obtains its goal by resorting to the use of heterogeneous elements that are foreign to the body.[5]

THE ANTHROPOSOPHICAL MEDICINE OF RUDOLF STEINER

Spiritual forces are imprisoned as if
by a spell in the substance of metal.

RUDOLF STEINER

Like Paracelsus, this great scholar from the beginning of the twentieth century, who conceived and founded anthroposophical medicine, granted importance to the correspondences between the cosmos and matter, between the elements of the earth and sky and our bodies. And the First Peoples, the Ancients of every tradition, say essentially the same thing—that is to say, that everything is interdependent, that we cannot consider ourselves as separate from the rest of the universe and even less so from our own earth and what it carries, for we are as intimately related to it as we are to our own cells.

THE KOLISKO EXPERIMENT

All of this comes from a certain assertion made by Rudolf Steiner at one of his conferences: "So long as matter remains in a solid state, it is subject to the forces of the earth. But once it moves into a liquid state, it undergoes the influence of the planets."

The eminent biologist L. Kolisko then had the idea for a series of experiments[6] that she went on to perform in 1920. Her question: How do aqueous solutions of metal salts behave in connection with the planets to which they are alleged to correspond?

The experiment was simple: She prepared metal salt solutions consisting of 1 gram of salt per 100 cubic centimeters of distilled water. She then poured 10 cc of this solution into a cup and placed vertically into the cup a loosely rolled paper filter. The solution was thereby "aspirated" by the filter paper, forming various "drawings" or images through the capillary action of the paper as it absorbed the solution. She repeated this simple experiment hundreds of times under the different aspects of the planets concerned through the play of correspondences. For example: gold chloride for the Sun, silver nitrate for the Moon, tin chloride for Jupiter, and so forth. She was able to observe that the drawings created in this way testified to actual planetary influences affecting the migration of the metals: The images were very precise before and after a phenomenon and non-existent while it was taking place.* They were clearly witnesses to cosmic forces that Mrs. Kolisko poetically called the "language of the stars."

These experiments permit the following observations:[7]

- Regularly and without fail the expected changes of the images left by the metallic salts on the filter paper occurred at the same times as celestial phenomena and only at those times.
- The duration of celestial events extends beyond what we can perceive.

During a solar eclipse, "it is chaos . . . several forces struggling to ensure their supremacy."†

The use of minerals in anthroposophical medicine is connected to these various correspondences and similarities. Minerals are used in the form of homeopathic distillations, more generally in the potency measured in decimals (whereas homeopathy primarily employs much higher dilutions: hundredths or more). It should be noted that in the majority of cases the plant-ingested form of the mineral is preferable to the pure mineral. Anthroposophical laboratories make their preparations according to certain natural laws so that the substance used will develop its maximum energy.

THE DE-CHELATED LITHOTHERAPY OF DR. TÉTAU AND DR. BERGERET

Lithotherapy uses the ore rather than the metals that are extracted from it. Offered in the form of drinkable phials (in 8X), these minerals are

---

*A colloidal metal solution created patterns on the paper that followed the waxing and waning of a particular planetary influence upon the earth. The images were the result of the effects of the planetary energy on its corresponding mineral.

† Because there are several planetary energies involved, no clear pattern can be discerned; the energies are too closely intermixed, resulting in a kind of chaos.

PRINCIPAL MINERALS USED IN DE-CHELATING LITHOTHERAPY

Adulaire	Lazulite
Apatite	Lepidolite
Auriferous Chalcopyrite	Lithic Tourmaline
Azurite	Mica Phlogopite
Barytine	Monazite
Beryl	Obsidian
Betafite	Orpiment
Blende	Pyrolusite
Bornite	Pink Sandstone
Versailles Limestone	Polar Magnetite
Celestine	Quadratic Feldspar
Conglomerat	Rhodonite
Diopside	Saccaroidal Marble
Garnerite	Sodalite
Glauconie	Stibine
Green Jasper	Trachite
Hematite	Ulexite
Iron Pyrite	

similar to colloidal mineral solutions. This therapeutic method has as its foundation rocks and minerals that have been diluted and potentized according to Hahnemann's method (that is, following the principles of homeopathy). It is a mineral therapy whose purpose is the treatment of patients through the administering of metals and metalloids. A nontoxic therapy, it acts on the "internal cellular environment of the patient and aims to normalize metabolic circuits that are disordered by a blockage on the enzymatic level."[8]

Pathological disorders connected to an enzymatic deficit have two essential causes:

- A total absence in the body of the crucial enzyme
- A deactivation of the necessary enzyme, which is present but not operative due to the failure or absence of the metallic ion that is required to activate it

Outside of cases of proven mineral deficiency, it happens that the body, under the effect of food or medicinal pollution, is not able to use the ions it needs, which then find themselves blocked, chelated, imprisoned. It is therefore necessary to unblock these ions by dechelating them. The use of Hahnemann-inspired metal dilutions allows for this release to occur. To accomplish this, minerals and natural rocks are used rather than the isolated chemical substance—thereby following Hahnemann's precepts, which have since been affirmed by research involving identifying the similarity between the crystalline structure of the mineral and that of the chelate from which the blocked metallic ion must be freed.

The basic principles explored in this chapter are the same as those at play in the use of colloidal minerals: the importance of a natural (plant or marine) source of the mineral, the mineral's ability to be assimilated, the importance of dilute concentrations, and the advantages of a complex intake that covers all our needs.

2

A HEALTHY DIET IS THE ESSENTIAL FOUNDATION OF OVERALL GOOD HEALTH

In the future, we will not be able to rely anymore on our premise that the consumption of a varied balanced diet will provide all the essential trace elements, because such a diet will be very difficult to obtain for millions of people.

DR. WALTER MERTZ,
U.S. DEPARTMENT OF AGRICULTURE
STATEMENT TO CONGRESS, 1977

Where can we find the minerals and nutrients that are essential to our health and longevity? In principle the source would be our diet, which basically consists of plant and animal products (with the animals' diet consisting of the same plants as ours). This is because, by drawing from the air the carbon necessary to manufacture the chains from which vitamins, amino acids, and essential fatty acids are synthesized, plants should be able to provide a large part of the nutrients we need. In order to meet our daily needs, however, it is necessary not only that we consume some twenty different vegetables in the proper proportions, but that these vegetables have been grown in soil that is sufficiently rich in nutrients and free from poisoning by the many different chemical products that are now in common use. As we shall see, it has become fairly difficult to meet these criteria. But the fact remains: *We cannot live without minerals and we will live wretchedly if we suffer from a mineral deficiency.*

Numerous epidemiological studies have provided ample proof that regular consumption of fruits and vegetables is essential for the prevention of a large number of debilitating diseases such as diabetes, cancer, cardiovascular disorders, and so on. These illnesses are particularly common in Western countries whose inhabitants eat too much fat, sugar, salt, and animal products and too few of the indispensable food fiber, vitamins, minerals, and other micronutrients necessary for our health.

We have moved far beyond the time when the human diet was regarded simply as a source of proteins, glucids, and lipids. The quality of food and its richness in micronutrients are now finally beginning to become a focus, even on the official level. This is particularly true of fruits and vegetables, especially when they are grown organically on healthy soils that are not depleted of essential elements. This is especially important given that plant-based products are particularly rich in bio-available antioxidants. The term *bio-available* refers to a substance that occurs in a form that is easily utilized by the body. We are currently aware of the major role played by antioxidants in the fight against premature aging and in the prevention of a large number of diseases. The benefits of these micronutrients point to the importance of having them, and those like them, at our body's disposal in such a way that they are completely harmless in nature and can act in complete synergy to protect the body's cellular environment.

Today there is much discussion about vitamins, which actually enjoy good press. But while vitamins are indeed necessary, the daily intake of the appropriate quantity of good quality minerals is equally important for our health. Minerals help regulate the body's elimination functions and help regenerate the blood on the molecular level, because of the way they bond with many of the body's enzymes. If we do not receive the proper amounts of the necessary minerals, we run a risk of living with chronic toxicity, which will bring about a chronic state of exhaustion.

"Minerals are the blood of our life," Ann Wigmore writes.[1] This has been true since the time eons past when the minerals of the ancient oceans combined with amino acids and enzymes to first create life forms. In fact, mineral salts are the very foundation of all life. Simultaneously present in the mineral, plant, and animal realms, mineral salts are responsible for the transfer of the energy running through all their substances and organisms.

It has long been thought that the variety and abundance of the modern diet was enough to prevent any risk of nutrient deficiency. We now know, however, that there is no factual basis for this assumption.

THE EXAMPLE OF CALCIUM

We have only to turn on the television during a commercial break to hear advertisers repeat that children, adults, and the elderly need calcium, and that women who have gone through menopause especially require it to avoid the risk of developing osteoporosis. These assertions bring great joy to the manufacturers of dairy products, who play a fairly prominent role in this kind of advertising, which has arrived at some conclusions that are currently hotly debated. Everyone agrees that the human body needs calcium to build a resistant skeleton, particularly during the growing years and as we enter older age, but the promoters of this information neglect to specify which kind of calcium (there are at least six different categories) is truly beneficial to our health. People, then, tend to take a little calcium as "fortification," but soon shelve the practice when the results of this therapy seem mediocre.

So what is the point of taking mineral supplements? We are told ceaselessly that our basic diet contains all the nutrients we need to enjoy good health—but are also told of the benefits of taking supplements such as calcium. Is our diet sufficiently nutrient rich? What would the reason be, then, for the obvious deterioration of health and the steep rise in degenerative diseases such as cancer, cardio-vascular diseases, and so forth, in the so-called developed nations? And what of the constant decrease in the human immune system's effectiveness, which engenders new pathologies and encourages the return of old scourges we had believed to be long eradicated?

It is easy to believe that one gets enough minerals in various forms, even from drinking mineral waters that contain large amounts of these nutrients, such as those high in calcium Yet as some readers may recall, there was a time when water with calcium was the target of heavy criticism. All kinds of harmful effects, including primarily kidney stones, were attributed to it, resulting in a plethora of water softeners, filters, and other systems intended to render tap water calcium-free or calcium-reduced. Now, however, the ads all around us maintain that just the opposite is true and promote a large array of hard waters—dressed up in this instance with the descriptive phrase "rich in calcium."

Yet I remain convinced that the calcium in hard water is no easier for our body to absorb than what we'd find in a piece of chalk. And even if the calcium in such water was present in the form of more easily absorbed calcium ions, in order for these to be used effectively by the body, we must have present an entire cocktail of other metal ions—notably, trace elements.

Furthermore, as you may well have grasped already, it is not only calcium and magnesium that we need (though a deficiency of the key mineral magnesium is in itself enough to create numerous disorders). The fact remains that in order to function well our body, just like that of all plants and animals, needs a balanced and sufficient quantity of all this planet's minerals in a form that can be absorbed and assimilated.

Too Much Milk? Too Many Dairy Products?

While efforts prompt us to drink more milk and consume more dairy products—whether they are in the form of yogurts, ricotta, and all kinds of cheeses, not to mention creamy desserts like flans, rice puddings, and ice cream (the list is endless)—it is not obvious that this is good for us. Quite the contrary.

While a baby, obviously, needs milk, it is clearly the milk of his or her mother—and not cow's milk (transformed for this purpose into formula) that will never have the virtues of breast milk—that is consumed without any intermediaries or transformations!

Cow's milk is designed for calves, just as the milk of each species of mammal has been intended by nature to cover the specific needs of its young. Only we humans have come up with the ludicrous notion that the milks of different mammals are interchangeable when in truth they are nothing of the sort.

Further, in nature adults are never seen drinking the milk produced by the female members of their respective species. Yet, while adult humans do not drink human breast milk, we drink cow's milk, just as children do. Could it be a kind of latent infantilism in our societies that compels this uninterrupted use? Ironically, the milk we drink is taken from mother cows that are then no longer able to provide their own calves with nourishment. These calves are bottle fed sterilized and irradiated cow's milk! Is there any wonder that our farm animals are in such a wretched state of health today? They are increasingly susceptible to all sorts of modern diseases that are evidently linked to their weak immune systems, which are the result of being deprived of their mothers' milk. As with humans, milk consumed directly from the mother breast—which prevents any loss of its vitamins, enzymes, and vital energy—contains a large quantity of antibodies intended to preserve the health of the calf and allow its immune system to fully mature. Thus the milk we drink, taken out of its natural context in unnatural conditions, taken from animals "forced" to produce in ever-larger quantities, is hardly the ideal food it is touted to be.

Like human breast milk, cow's milk contains calcium, but in dosages appropriate for the needs of small calves, not human beings. As Anne Laroche-Walter has shown in her excellent book *Lait de vache, blancheur trompeuse* (Cow's Milk, Deceptively White),[2] despite its richness in calcium, cow's milk does in fact encourage mineral loss in humans because its lack of the specific ossein for humans (the organic basis of bone tissue) makes it hard for our bodies to retain minerals—the complete opposite of what we might expect. Furthermore, the phosphorus-calcium ratio in cow's milk is not suitable for humans; an excess of phosphorus carries the threat of insufficient calcification. The proportion of the two determines how readily usable each mineral is. In addition, the lactic acid found in milk and commercially prepared dairy products is levrogyric, which contributes to the elimination of our body's calcium. (Only a dextrogyric* lactic acid—such as that found in whey manufactured traditionally without the addition of pressure—helps our body to retain calcium.)

Levrogyric (meaning "clockwise") and *dextrogyric* (meaning "counterclockwise") refer to the direction of the spiral of the acid molecule, which in turn determines its acid/alkaline balance.

Finally, all of the calcium from cow's milk that remains unassimilated by the body accumulates in certain tissues and organs, where it can cause cysts, various kinds of stones, osteoarthritis, and minor calcification. It has long been noted that it is impossible to cure the decalcification or osteoarthritis of a person who drinks milk.

NO, OUR DIET DOES NOT MEET OUR NEEDS!

Even eating the varied diet recommended to us will generally not give us the elements our body needs to function in an optimal manner. Our body is like a car: It needs gas, oil, and water in order for its motor to function properly.

But the warning bell about this state of affairs was already sounded close to seventy years ago.

In 1936 a report from the United Sates Senate (U.S. Senate Document 264, 74th Congress, Second Session) tried to draw attention to this serious problem, but apparently inspired no reactions. Its words, however, were quite clear and its conclusions striking. See appendix 1 (page 177) for extracts from this significant document that highlight its essential points, which are summarized below:

Virgin and cultivated lands alike are seriously deficient in minerals and the grains, fruits, vegetables, and beans harvested from these depleted soils in turn exhibit a mineral deficiency—and finally, those who eat them will incur serious mineral deficiencies, with all the well-known adverse consequences for their health. The sole means of preventing and curing these pathological states is by taking mineral and nutritional supplements.

As John Hamaker and Donald Weaver suggest in their book *Survival of Civilization,* we may understand precisely "why everything living on earth has reached a point of slow death by starvation . . . The quality (health, vigor, intelligence, longevity, and so on) of every living organism depends on the protoplasm of life in the soil, which is itself dependent upon the availability of mineral elements from rock."[3]

Every time plants are harvested, a large portion of the soil's minerals is stripped away. Now because of the intensive use for many years of organophosphate and potassium fertilizers intended to increase crop yields, the situation is far from being improved. Regarding the health of

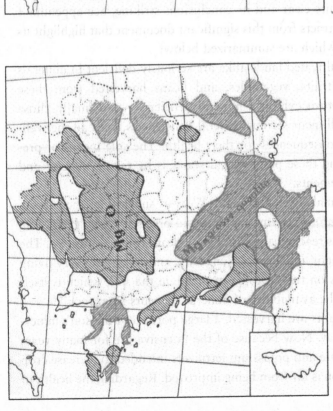

Magnesium Distribution in France (Source: Based on a map published by the French Ministry of Public Works)

   Little if any magnesium in the soil

   Large amounts of magnesium in the soil (generally from dolomite)

Distribution of observable cancer in France (Source: Based on statistics from individual arrondissements, or townships, of less than 5,000 inhabitants)

   Coefficients greater than 8.5, equaling a large incidence of cancer (60 arrondissements)

   Coefficients less than 3.5, equaling few cases of cancer (102 arrondissements)

Fig. 2.1. Maps showing the results of L. Robinet's geographical study correlating regions in France that are deficient in magnesium in the soil and regions where a significant number of cancer cases had been observed. Reproduced from Politique préventive du cancer by Pierre Delbet (Paris: Éditions Denoël, 1944).

our soil, we can all imagine how much we must adjust its condition for the nearly seven decades that have elapsed since the report to the U.S. Congress was published. The report itself supplies evidence that information essential to our survival and our health was known and widely studied—but how was it smothered? Why did it take so many years to relaunch these ideas and attempt to act on them? It is evident that the crises we are experiencing today were already visible on the horizon decades ago. If these warnings had been heeded then, perhaps we might have avoided arriving at the critical state we have reached today as a result of our need to always have more.

MAGNESIUM DEFICIENCY AND CANCER

In France similar research has been undertaken and similar conclusions have been reached. One researcher, Professor Pierre Delbet, expressed a fervent wish that one day the Ministry of Agriculture would merge with the Ministry of Health, given the obvious effects the actions of the former have on the latter. His research focused primarily on the importance of magnesium salts (most of all, magnesium chloride) in animal and human health.[4]

Born in 1861, Pierre Delbet was considered an "eminent authority" as a result of an exemplary medical career of more than thirty years. He served as a hospital intern and a senior hospital lecturer, graduated from medical school and went on to become a surgeon, was awarded prizes on several occasions by the Sorbonne Medical School and the Medical Academy, of which he was a member, and authored several books that became the voices of authority in their fields. He departed this world in 1957 at the age of ninety-seven. All of this is to show that he was by no means a quack or charlatan. Nevertheless, new ideas like his are rarely given the welcome they deserve, especially in the medical profession.

It was during Delbet's time that the rapid increase in the occurrence of cancer in the Western nations had become a subject of great concern. It was an ideal moment for verifying the truth of his theory: that magnesium deficiency was the culprit in this increase. Any noticeable reduction in the magnesium intake among the inhabitants of these Western countries might explain the sudden outbreak of different cancers.

The result of Delbet's research in this field focused on three essential causes of magnesium deficiency: the bolting of flour, the refining of salt, and the weak magnesium content of fruits and vegetables.

> Everything that lives is a product of the soil and retains some part of its chemical constitution. So wouldn't our diet and consequently the soil be the logical places to seek out the reason for either the frequency or rarity of cancer?[5]

According to Delbert, when the soil is depleted of magnesium (which is both the natural condition of the soil in certain regions and is also a result of forced or intensive farming methods), it will be accompanied by flourishing cancer rates. Hence the value of mineral fertilizers—one aspect of Delbet's cancer prevention policy—which ensure a sufficient input of magnesium (ground silicate rocks, natural phosphates, lithothamnia, maerl, dolomites, natural magnesium sulfate, and so on).

DID YOU KNOW?

Ten years of intensive farming is all it takes to completely deplete the soil of all its minerals.

As it happens, this problem is not solely the prerogative of the West; profoundly depleted soils can be found throughout the entire world.

It should be remembered that this research was performed at the beginning of the last century. Its importance for our time resides in the fact that it was then still possible to demonstrate parameters such as a soil's deficiency of magnesium and its repercussions on health. Today this is almost impossible, for the majority of our arable surfaces are in a state of almost complete depletion. The problem of magnesium deficiency in humans remains, however, accompanied by all the additional causes of illness that our polluted environment abundantly furnishes. It is no longer cause for surprise to see cancer cases multiplying everywhere and in all age groups, even among the most young.

These were the conclusions reached by Pierre Delbet:

The surveys made several years ago concerning the geographical distribution of cancer have shown that vast regions of the globe are almost unscathed by this plague, whereas others are sorely afflicted by it. The proportional differences are so great that the connection between cancer and where you live is beyond doubt; they range from differences of 1 to 10, 12, and even 14.[6]

To prove this, geographical studies were undertaken and published in 1929 by L. Robinet in order to see if the geological maps of regions poor in magnesium coincided with those of regions where a significant number of cancer cases had been observed. According to Delbet: "The comparison of the two maps was gripping. They were identical!" The same research was carried out in other countries with the same results. For example, in Egypt and Tunisia, where the food was particularly rich in magnesium because of the high content of that element in the soil and in the water, no cancers were found.

If the foods were deficient in magnesium, it was determined that, even at that early date, it was due to the low levels of this element (and of all the other nutrients) in the vegetables and fruits grown by means of intensive farming methods on depleted soils. As most people are well aware, the world's soils have not improved since the time of these first studies. Today it is all too obvious that the same situation is a reality: Our food is wanting magnesium and all the other minerals that our daily diet should be supplying us.

3
THE IMPORTANCE
OF SOIL QUALITY

Certainly the depletion of our soil is not the sole reason for the lack of nutrients in the foods we eat. Our cooking methods, for example, also strip our foods of a large portion of vitamins and minerals (many of which can be found in the cooking water that collects on our plates or gets left in the pot). The deficiencies in canned foods and other highly processed products from the food industry are even more severe.

The soil, however, is where the problem begins. Because they are unable to synthesize minerals, plants must draw these substances from the soil. This is why the condition of the soil on earth is of the utmost importance. If it is depleted—which is frequently the case today—our fruits and vegetables will be devoid of these minerals and we will have none of them to consume.

This underscores how seriously we need to care for the land in which our food is grown. When the ground is exhausted of its minerals, the harvests it produces are also deficient in essential nutrients. Ultimately, in a kind of poetic justice, the weakening of the earth leads to our own ill health.

The status of mineral levels in foods is not a mystery; the color and flavor of fresh foods reflect the mineral values of the soil in which they were grown and thus these values in the foods themselves.

Few people would even dream of comparing a tomato grown in a garden with naturally rich soil and picked in the middle of the summer

ONE EXAMPLE:
MODERN FLOUR AND MODERN CARROTS

According to recent analyses, during the past 40 years white flour has lost 16 percent of its selenium, 48 percent of its molybdenum, 60 percent of its calcium, 68 percent of its copper, 71 percent of its phosphorus, 77 percent of its potassium, 78 percent of its zinc, 85 percent of its magnesium, 86 percent of its manganese, 89 percent of its cobalt, and 98 percent of its chromium. As for carrots, which were once a wonderful source of magnesium, those that can be found in the supermarket produce section have only a trace of this important element.

To make a bad situation worse, even when our soil is "reconverted," it has relatively little in common with perfectly healthy soil, such as the kind in which the luxuriant forests of our ancestors grew. Our farmlands would need to be left fallow for decades, along with being constantly enriched with organic ingredients such as compost and decayed cover crops, to recover their former properties and, in return, provide us with food worthy of the name.

The first line of defense in the prevention of nutritional deficiencies thus involves defense of the soil and the restoration of its humus, that rich, organic portion of the soil resulting from the partial decomposition of plant matter. This strategy is all the more imperative as the rapid growth of livestock ranching necessitates grazing practices that impoverish the soil on vast tracts of land. The use of chemical fertilizers on our ever-larger corporate and factory farms causes the situation to deteriorate even more. For example, excess potassium leads to greater deficiencies of magnesium and excess ammonia from fertilizers is responsible for deficiencies of copper. It is easy to see why there are now sound arguments for seeking other forms of natural minerals that are easy for the body to assimilate.

at the peak of its ripeness to one purchased in a supermarket in the month of January—even when, in order to perfect the illusion and fool the consumer, the supermarket tomato has been genetically modified and colored so as to appear as if it were perfectly ripe and picked the evening before.

But is soil even necessary? There are certainly "benefits" (for whom?) in today's soil-less agriculture that makes it possible to grow fruits and vegetables on an artificial substrate without any need for the plants to ever touch the ground. Even the sun is no longer indispensable; quality artificial grow lights that mimic the sun's warmth and light are now available. What these technological advances truly mean, however, is that we may say goodbye to the nutritional and revitalizing qualities that are supposed to come from the foods we eat.

"THE SOIL MAKES THE ANIMAL"

Never before has this ancient saying been more true. Of course, intensive agriculture does increase yields, and sometimes even several harvests a season, depending on the farming methods and region. Yet because of inevitable soil exhaustion, farmers are forced to turn to chemical fertilizers and pesticides of all kinds to successfully grow their crops. Rather than providing the soil and the plants growing in it with proper and complete nourishment, these fertilizers generally contain only nitrogen, phosphorus, and potassium to simply increase production to the maximum amount possible. Providing these limited nutrients is equivalent to meeting a growing child's nutritional needs by supplying him or her with nothing but standard calcium tablets. Soil requires exactly what the human body requires: a natural *cocktail* of all minerals in their proper proportion.

> Most farmers use chemical fertilizers and pesticides routinely to produce lush crops. These fertilizers generally contain only nitrogen, phosphorus, and potassium (NPK) because that is all the plant requires to produce a maximum crop yield. Typically, chemical phosphates (rather than the much needed organic phosphorus mineral) are added to soil for growing fruits and vegetables. Now these chemical products destroy the tiny microorganisms in the soil that are necessary to convert inorganic minerals into a usable form for the plant to

absorb. Not only is the soil already lacking naturally occurring minerals, but it is difficult for the plants to assimilate what minerals are left. Plants will grow in soil that is low in minerals and trace elements such as magnesium, manganese, iron, iodine, chromium, and selenium. However these minerals and trace elements are of vital importance to humans; therefore the lack of them in the diet can result in severe deficiency diseases.[1]

When Mount Saint Helens erupted in May 1980, the apple producers in the states of Oregon and Washington were in great despair because the thick layer of volcanic ash that covered their land completely wiped out their harvests. But the following year, their apples grew twice as large as before and their trees bore more fruit than they ever had. The fact is that the fine powder of ash was extremely rich in trace elements, which completely reinvigorated the mineral content of the soil.

THE FLAVOR OF FRUITS AND VEGETABLES DEPENDS ON THEIR MINERAL CONTENT

A common observation today is that while the fruits and vegetables that are grown are beautiful in appearance, they have lost the flavor they once had. Those who cultivate their own gardens in soil that is rich and who follow the rules of organic farming or those who purchase produce that is grown in this way can appreciate the now rare, superior flavor of products that are cultivated with respect for the earth and its balance. But in addition to enjoying the delicious flavor of such fruits and vegetables, they also are reaping a harvest in health. It just so happens that there is a close connection between flavor and wealth in minerals: The fewer the minerals, the weaker the flavor.

Organic farmers who cultivate their land through the use of natural fertilizers certainly avoid the disastrous problems that come with chemical fertilizers and dangerous pesticides. But because cultivation of any kind depletes the minerals and nutrients in the soil and because plants do not have the ability to synthesize minerals, ultimately the organic farmer's produce will not be any more nutritious than produce grown following standard commercial practice. Any soil under cultivation requires that its minerals and nutrients be restored regularly.

We may wonder how ancient peoples who did not have the benefit of fertilizers handled this problem, or how contemporary peoples who live off their harvest alone—like the Hunza of Pakistan—address this issue. It is worth noting that great ancient civilizations such as those of the Egyptians, the Chinese, and the Indians always developed near large rivers (in this case, the Nile, the Yellow River, and the Ganges, respectively). These regions were flooded annually during the winter months, and during this time tons upon tons of rock, mud, and earth from mountains located at a considerable distance upstream would spill over the rivers' flood plains and enrich the arable lands. It is easy to see why ancient peoples prayed to their gods to bring the annual floods—though today we pray for precisely the opposite! This cyclical inundation brought the earth the minerals it needed and thus led to harvests of high quality grains and produce.

4
POLLUTION: THE HEAVY TRIBUTE EXACTED BY MODERN LIFE

All the medical research and billions of dollars spent to find cures have not altered the advance of killer diseases. Perhaps it is because our soil is still mineral-deficient and our bodies are constantly bombarded with toxins found in the food we eat, the air we breathe and the water we drink. A body that is not receiving optimum nutrition cannot effectively deal with these toxins that poison and weaken the immune system. We must look to full-spectrum nutritional supplementation to prevent premature aging [and] disease and to experience optimum health.

TONITA D'RAYE

Minerals and trace elements, essential to a healthy metabolism, have become even more precious because of the numerous deficiencies that are caused by the stresses and disruptions of modern life. It seems that we should never have trouble meeting our mineral needs, for these essential elements can be found in the food we eat and the water we drink. And yet . . .

For millennia our ancestors followed a simple lifestyle characterized by cooperation with nature, but in the space of a few centuries modern humans have relinquished this lifestyle in exchange for one that is radically different. And in the last few decades, as a result of overwhelming technological advances, we have been drawn even farther away from our natural environment, with consequences that we are only now truly beginning to grasp. We have enjoyed the benefits of modern society, but are paying a price that grows higher and higher.

The air we breathe is polluted—particularly by the toxins from exhaust. The dust from various pollutants settles at a rate of about 2 grams per square foot in an apartment located in a city. In rural areas this figure is usually no higher than 0.9 mg! To clean up our air, it is estimated that the equivalent of 800,000 freight cars a day would be required to carry away all the impurities that are removed!

Our air is not the only portion of our world that is in crisis, however. The planet's water is in a catastrophic state. Many rivers are so polluted that they can no longer cleanse themselves—a drastic change from even the time of my childhood, when it was still safe to play freely in our rivers and lakes. Our oceans are in no better condition. Some twenty years ago Jacques Cousteau reported that 40 percent of aquatic life had already been destroyed by the poisons that had been discharged into the ocean. Every year we spill into the sea more than 5,000 tons of mercury; 5,000 tons of lead; 100,000 tons of pesticides and PCBs; and 10,000,000 tons of petroleum. And these are only a few of the highly toxic products that make their way into the earth's water.

The earth that carries and feeds us is exhausted and poisoned, and the toxins we spread over it eventually make their way back to us. According to a German study by W. Heupke, on a daily basis we absorb some 4 grams of dangerous—or at the least, questionable—chemicals in the foods we eat in the form of heavy metals, chemical fertilizers, pesticides, PVCs, and radioactive substances. To get a full picture of this problem, we must note that the different pesticides alone number more than 4,000, which are applied at an average of 5 kilograms per hectare of land (translating to an average of 1 kilogram per person). These products are stored in our fatty tissue and take years to decompose to harmless levels. In the meantime, they can wreak havoc on our enzymatic and nervous systems.

Here is what Dr. Americo Mosca, winner of the famous prize in chemistry at the Brussels World's Fair, had to say as early as 1974:

> I calculate that in the United States the use of toxic genetic chemicals
> (herbicides, insecticides, hormones, steroids, etc.) causes damage equal
> to atomic fallout from 145 H-bombs of 14 megatons each or, in terms

SOME SURPRISING FIGURES*

- The application of chemical fertilizers world-wide has risen from 7,000,000 tons in 1945 to 150,000,000 tons today.
- Of the pesticides we can trace in our food, 90 percent are found in animal products and less than 10 percent appear in plant products.
- 97 percent of the varieties of vegetables that were customarily included on the United States Department of Agriculture's list in the 1940s have disappeared.
- 80 percent of factory farm animals are in poor health.
- 5 plant species are permanently lost every day.

* From *Soignez-vous*, April 6, 2002, and Lucy and Soly Fabiana de Oliveira, *Tous végétariens demain* (Ibis Rouge Éditions, 2002).

of atomic bombs, from 72,500 atomic bombs of the type dropped on Hiroshima. For this reason in the United States in the last ten years disease of all kinds and births of mentally retarded babies have increased tremendously. The damage to plants, crops, soil fertility, and water pollution are practically incalculable. If use of these toxic genetic chemicals persists in agriculture . . . it will cause the destruction of the American people.[1]

PERMANENT POISONING

At first glance it would appear that we receive only a small dose of all these poisons from the air we breath, the water we drink, and the foods we eat. If we consider, however, that the surface area of our body is a little more than 2 square meters, that the surface area of our lungs is 100 square meters, and the surface area of both our small and large intestine is about 2000 square meters, it is easier to see how even small doses of toxins could have serious consequences. As Sigmund Schmidt emphasized as early as 1974 in a book entitled *Can We Protect Our Bodies from the Poisons in the Surrounding Environment?*,[2] in the span of 30 years the average human being consumes more than 4,000 gallons of liquid (900 of which are milk; 2,000 of which are tea and coffee; and 1,100 of which are wine, beer, and other kinds of alcoholic beverages); about 40,000 pounds of potatoes, vegetables, bread, grains, and so forth; and 6,000 pounds of fish and even more than that of meat. An individual also inhales some 4,000,000 gallons of air (in a 24-hour period, a person breathes 12 cubic meters of air!) and, if a smoker, smokes some 200,000 cigarettes with some 10 pounds of tar that will burden his or her respiratory tract (and that of those who are in his or her proximity, although in lesser amounts).

We should add that when they are combined, environmental toxins have the vexing property of strengthening each other to such an extent that they are forty times more toxic to a developing fetus than to the mother. In addition, they remain stored in the body for years, which enables them to penetrate the body's 200 billion cells and seriously damage them by, among other tactics, obstructing cellular respiration and countering various processes of synthesis.

Over the course of the last fifty years the number of these polluting chemical substances has grown tremendously. For the more than 5,000,000 chemical products listed as available in the year 1990, 20,000 to 27,000 were considered carcinogenic.

5
WE SHOULD ALL LIVE
FOR 120 TO 140 YEARS

We know that all higher mammals have an average life span—between the time of birth and natural death—that is approximately equal to seven times the time it takes them to grow to maturity.

Dogs, for example, require almost two years to grow to full maturity, which gives them a longevity of 12 to 14 years. The only exceptions to this are humans, who rarely even attain 100 years of age today, which amounts to merely five times their growth period. During Napoleon's time in France, despite a lower overall average life expectancy due to many factors that were then in play, there were always at least ten or fifteen people at any one time who had reached the age of at least 115 years. Although the average life expectancy has increased since that time and continues to grow, the number of people exhibiting such longevity has decreased dramatically so that it is now quite rare that anyone lives to such an age.

Our genetic potential should in fact allow us to live at the minimum 120 years. Of course, in order to achieve such longevity we must nourish our body's cells appropriately. Witness the Hunzas, the people who live in eastern Pakistan and whose longevity has become the stuff of legend.

REMARKABLE LONGEVITY

A case has been recorded of one man living on the Tibetan border who was born in 1677 and who was awarded a certificate from the Chinese emperor on the occasion of his 150th birthday. He was awarded another certificate when he turned 200, and another when he reached the age of 250. It is said that he died at the age of 256.

A number of the world's peoples have beaten the records for longevity—as long as they have continued to follow their traditional lifestyles. Among these are, in the eastern hemisphere, the Georgians, the Armenians, the Abkhasians, and the people of Azerbeijan, and on the opposite side of the world the Vilkabamba Indians of Ecuador and the indigenous peoples living around Lake Titicaca in Peru.

National Geographic, known for its quality, factual reporting, has often cited records of longevity noted around the world. An article in the January 1973 edition looks specifically at those who had lived beyond 100 years of age. Included in the article is a photo of an Armenian man harvesting tea leaves in the Caucasus. After verifying his birth certificate, baptismal certificate, and other official documents, as well as those of his children, it was determined that he was 167 years old.*

Another photo accompanying the article shows a 136-year-old woman, also from the Caucasus, holding a cigar in one hand and a glass of vodka in the other at a celebration of the one-hundredth wedding anniversary of two friends!

Similarly, the Guinness Book of World Records cites a Syrian man who died at the age of 133 after having married for the fourth time at the age of 80 and fathering nine children from this marriage, a statistic that indicates that he was fathering children after he had turned 100—a feat that is most noteworthy at a time when male fertility rates are threatened.

---

*From Joel D. Wallach, Dead Doctors Don't Lie: Learn Why the Average Life Span of an M.D. Is only 58 Years! (Wellness Publications, 1999).

GLACIER'S MILK:
THE ELIXIR OF LONG LIFE?

The people of the five different cultures mentioned in these examples who live for 120 to 140 years of age share a specific common denominator: They spend their lives in villages perched on the glacial lands of the high mountains at altitudes that vary from 8000 to 14,500 feet. The climate is quite dry in these regions, with average rainfall in the neighborhood of 1/2 inch or less per year and with little snow and dew. In the areas where all of these communities exist, glaciers eat away the mountain rock at the rate of several fractions of an inch each year. As a result of this process, glacier's milk—which is simply the water that has melted from the glaciers—contains some 60 to 72 different minerals, depending on the region. Unlike popular mineral waters sold in stores today, this melt-off from beneath the glaciers is not clear. In fact, it looks like milk with a yellowish or bluish tint—which is what earned this liquid its name, whether it comes from Tibet or the region around Lake Titicaca. Not only have the people of these regions consumed this "milk" for some 2,500 to 5,000 years, but they also use it to water their crops and have been irrigating their fields with it for millennia—with the result that the mineral content of their lands is continually replenished and the nutritional value of the food they grow is exceptionally high. The people who live in these high mountain villages enjoy astounding health and energy. Heart problems are almost unheard of, as are cancer, high blood pressure, glaucoma, birth defects, hyperactivity in children, learning disabilities, diabetes, arthritis, osteoporosis, cataracts, obesity, and many of the other ills that plague our culture. All of this, it seems, is tied to the colloidal minerals that are abundant in their glacial water.

We now know that the minerals present in the plants we eat govern our cellular metabolism and are essential for maintaining good health and preventing disease. Everyone of us possesses the same genetic potential to enjoy robust health for 120 years or more. Each of us also holds the potential to reverse the process of premature aging, if we immediately start taking into account our true nutritional needs.

With regard to our own centenarians, the cause of death most prevalent among them is rarely a heart attack or some other physiological malfunction. Rather, fatality is largely due to a fall resulting in broken bones from which an elderly person has trouble recovering because of osteoporosis, the result of a nutritional deficiency of calcium, or from dehydration and the deficiencies that accompany it during the hottest months of the year.

MINERALS FOR LIVESTOCK, MEDICATIONS FOR HUMANS

I recently had the opportunity to read the particularly sharp-toned transcript of an address given at a conference by Dr. Joel Wallach, a veterinarian, naturopath, and Nobel nominee in medicine in 1991.[1] What interests him primarily is the importance of vitamins and minerals in human nutrition. This topic runs counter to what seems to be the current trend in conventional medicine, which is to shunt us onto the path of chemical prescriptions that are manipulated by pharmaceutical companies. Dr. Wallach's story is surprising.

His father was a farmer who raised veal for slaughter. He produced his own feed using his own grains and soy, which he ground together to make flour. He then added certain quantities of vitamins, minerals, and trace elements to this flour, which he then formed into pellets for his animals. When he was a child, Joel Wallach remarked to his father that no one in their house took any of these minerals and vitamins, yet livestock farmers considered them indispensable to the health of their calves. Upon entering the University of Missouri's School of Agriculture, Wallach's main courses of study were animal nutrition and soil conservation. After graduating he pursued veterinary medicine, in which he further observed that nutrition played a crucial role in the prevention and treatment of animal disease and was the sole means to making the raising of livestock a profitable venture.

After completing his education, he worked as a veterinarian specializing in the care and treatment of wild animals housed in zoos throughout the United States. At that time he was entrusted with the task of performing autopsies on the animals who had died of natural causes in zoos. He began to develop the idea of conducting a study on animals' particular sensitivities to various kinds of environmental pollution. Over the course of a dozen years, he performed more than 17,500 autopsies on more than 450 different species of animal. At the same time he also performed autopsies on more than 3,000 human beings who lived in close contact with zoos. This is what he discovered:

> All the animals and humans dead of natural causes were in fact dead of nutritional deficiencies . . . And we reached this conclusion during the autopsy by means of chemistry, biochemistry and what have you, as well as by simple visual observation on the autopsy table. I couldn't get over it.[2]

According to a World Health Organization study of 33 countries, the United States holds a sad record: One out of every 5,000 children in the United States is born with a birth defect or other congenital deformation.[3]

We can compare this with the incidence of birth defects among the livestock raised in the United States: An anomaly is found in 1 out of every 500,000 births.

As it happens, young calves intended for slaughter receive a daily food ration containing forty to fifty minerals—including zinc (a vital trace element that is essential to all metabolic processes, including the synthesis of DNA, the function and maturation of the reproductive organs, and protection against congenital defects)—whereas foods made specifically for babies contain at most twelve.

The discovery of these statistics compelled Wallach to write 75 scientific articles and several books, and to give interviews to more than 1,700 newspapers, magazines, radio stations and television stations in hopes of generating interest in these findings. But none materialized. To this he responded disarmingly, "After that there was only one thing left: . . . to go back to school and become a physician. I finally got a license to kill."[4]

After earning his medical degree, Wallach set up practice as a general practitioner in Portland, Oregon, where he applied to his human patients everything he had learned about animal nutrition. The results matched his expectations and served as the foundation for his later research on human nutrition and its ramifications on life expectancy.

Wallach spent a good part of his life establishing some interesting statistics, including this unusual observation: While the average life expectancy of people in general in the United States is 75.5 years, the average life span of doctors is only 58 years, which led him to the conclusion that to improve our life expectancy, we should not seek to study medicine! Other conclusions include this point to remember concerning nutrition: "We have a daily requirement of almost 103 basic nutrients, which consist of at least 72 minerals, 16 vitamins, 12 essential amino acids, and 3 essential fatty acids."[5]

If these nutrients are not provided to the body each day, we risk incurring a nutritional deficiency and all the adverse consequences that entails for health. As Dr. Wallach's studies indicated to him, the majority of people who seemed to have died of natural causes actually suffered from nutritional deficiencies.

6

SUPPORTING RESEARCH

There are quite a number of other interesting studies in the field of human nutrition that point to the importance of micro-nutrients to our overall health. Several of these are referred to in this chapter.

CANCER AND NUTRIENTS

The province of Hunan in China now has the highest cancer rate in the world. Recently, a study was completed there involving nutritional supplements: Test groups were given various minerals and vitamins at twice the recommended daily allowance (which is actually a fairly low amount). Thus one group received 120 mg of Vitamin C (note that the lowest-dose Vitamin C tablet is 500 mg and that Linus Pauling advised taking 10,000 mg a day as a way to avoid cancer), another group took zinc, another Vitamin E, and so forth. At this stage a clear result emerged for only one group: that which had been given a combination of Vitamin E, beta-carotene, and selenium. In this group a mortality rate reduction of 9 percent over five years was achieved—a considerable improvement over the standard mortality rate. For those people in the group suffering from cancer, particularly cancers of the stomach and esophagus, 21 percent survived as compared to the control group that did not receive Vitamin E, beta-carotene, and selenium. This improved result was obtained when only three basic nutrients in low doses were supplied to a test group—yet the human body requires close to one hundred nutrients every day.

ARTHRITIS AND THE
ROLE OF CHICKEN CARTILAGE

Today there is a very simple, effective, and inexpensive treatment for arthritis: powdered dried chicken cartilage—specifically, 1 teaspoonful in a glass of fruit juice once a day. Shark cartilage, which is quite rich in various nutrients, also works well in this application. According to a study performed by Harvard Medical School, arthritis sufferers who had previously been treated by conventional means with no results took this dosage of chicken cartilage and found that all pain and inflammation disappeared in ten days. In three months, they had recovered lasting mobility. The head researcher's analysis of the study's results states: "After three months, it was obvious that the medication displayed true effectiveness."[1] It is amusing to see that chicken cartilage, once proved to be effective, became a "medication." Yet there is nothing to stop any one of us from personally preparing this "medication." Chicken cartilage—which is essentially found at the soft ends of the bones—is simply dried in the oven, after which it is crushed enough to allow taking a teaspoonful every morning. Of course, the quality of the chicken is important: It is best to use one that was free range and raised on organic grain, and who exhibited no abnormal growth traits. The gelatin from animal bones has the same effect as that of cartilage, but ingesting this poses the threat of mad cow disease.

ALZHEIMER'S DISEASE
AND THE ROLE OF VITAMIN E

Only fifty years ago Alzheimer's Disease was still a rare condition. A similar condition evidencing the same brain lesions appeared in livestock but was treatable in its early stages with high doses of Vitamin E and vegetable oil. A recent study led by the University of California Medical School and published in July 1992 confirms what was taught fifty years ago in veterinary schools: "Vitamin E is effective against the memory disorders experienced by persons suffering from Alzheimer's disease." We might say, without being completely tongue in cheek, that it could be worthwhile to seek treatment from a veterinarian . . .

KIDNEY STONES AND
THE ROLE OF CALCIUM

If you are suffering from kidney stones, the first thing that your doctor will recommend is avoiding all foods containing calcium, including dairy products and nutritional supplements, because it is currently believed by some physicians that kidney stones are formed from the calcium that is absorbed through food. whereas the opposite is the case. In fact, kidney stones are formed from the calcium that our body frees from bones when it becomes necessary to balance a serious calcium deficiency—which is why many people with serious cases of osteoporosis also suffer from kidney stones. Once again, it is animal care that has guided our understanding. Veterinarians are taught that it is necessary to give calcium, magnesium, and boron to animals in order to prevent kidney stones.

A study directed by the Harvard Medical School in March 1993 declared that contrary to what has been thought, those who consume foods rich in calcium will see a considerable reduction in their risk of one day developing kidney stones. This study was based on the results collected from more than 45,000 individuals. It was also noted that those whose calcium levels were highest never suffered from urinary tract stones.

ANEURISMS AND VASCULAR
ACCIDENTS AND THE ROLE OF COPPER

Aneurisms and other disruptions of the cerebral vascular system are more and more common today and can strike at any age. An aneurism occurs when an artery becomes clogged and its elastic fibers become weak or distended. A 1957 study indicated a deficiency in copper caused aneurisms.

The pilot study focused on 250,000 turkeys and was followed up by studies on other livestock as well as rats and mice. This reveals the considerable implication of a copper deficiency in this pathology. For additional information on the connection between copper and aneurism, see *Prescription for Nutritional Healing: A to Z Guide to Supplements* by Phyllis A. Balch and James Balch (New York: Avery Publishing Group, 2002). The first symptom of this copper deficiency is the graying of the hair and the appearance of wrinkles, as well as varicose veins. All this can be traced back to a loss of flexibility in the body's elastic fibers.

MYOCARDIOPATHY AND
THE ROLE OF SELENIUM

Many studies have indicated that myocardiopathy, along with muscular deficiencies and other forms of myopathy, appear to have a connection to a deficiency in selenium.

HIGH BLOOD PRESSURE AND
THE ROLES OF SALT AND CALCIUM

Here we can turn again to Dr. Wallach:

What's the first nutritional thing your doctor will tell you to give up when you get high blood pressure? Salt. Everybody knows that one, it has been ingrained in our heads. Well, they must think we are dumber than cows, because what is the first thing you put out for your cows, and it's about that big? A salt block. No farmer is going to be economically viable if you don't put a salt block out for your livestock. They're going to die. They're going to get their veterinary bill and they are going to go crazy. Now we're supposed to believe that we don't need salt, that we can get everything we need out of your lettuce and your whole wheat bread, and stuff like that. Well don't believe that one either. If you believe that, I've got some more ocean front property in Montana. Remember, those long-lived people [the Hunza] put a big chunk of rock salt the size of a big black Concord grape in every cup of tea, and they drink about 40 cups of tea a day cause they live at high altitudes where it is very dry, and they have to keep hydrated. And they put butter in their tea. They put two pats of butter and chunks of rock salt. They don't put the pink stuff or the blue stuff, or skim milk, or Creamora, or whatever it is. Guess what? The doctors who lived to be 58 tell you, "No salt, no butter." The people who live to be 120, they put in butter and salt. You have got to make some choices.

They took 30 million dollars of your tax money, and two years ago, after a 20 year study, they came out and said that they took 5,000 people with high blood pressure [. . .] They took them off their medication, and put them on a reduced salt diet, a restricted salt diet, and they all died. No big surprise. But somebody got a Ph.D. degree and everybody was happy, right? But when they looked at this result, they said, "Oh, only 99.7% of the people didn't get any results from that before they died. 0.3% did get some results, dropped their blood pressure 1 point before they died, by restricting their salt." So the referees said, "Oh, doesn't matter. You might as well let high blood pressure patients eat salted peanuts, and dill pickles, and salt their food to taste, cause it doesn't matter. In fact, worrying about the salt is more stress than taking the salt."

Then they had a controlled group with 5,000 people with high blood pressure and they doubled their RDA [Recommended Daily Allowance] of calcium and they stopped their experiment in 6 weeks. Cause 85% of them were cured of their high blood pressure, just by doubling their calcium intake.[2]

INSOMNIA AND PMS AND THE ROLE OF CALCIUM

A recent study completed by the University of San Diego showed that simply taking twice the RDA of calcium is enough to ease most of the uncomfortable symptoms—both physical and emotional—of PMS. The same was also true for cases of insomnia, especially when associated with nocturnal leg discomfort.

LUMBAGO AND THE ROLE OF CALCIUM AND COPPER

Painful lumbago is generally linked to latent osteoporosis and thus to a deficiency in calcium. It has also been linked to a deficiency in copper, which results in a distension of the elastic fibers that maintain the alignment of the vertebra. Copper is needed to make adenosine triphosphate (ATP), the energy our body uses to function. Synthesis of some hormones requires copper, as does collagen (the "glue" that holds muscle tissue together) and tyrosinase (the enzyme responsible for skin pigmentation). Copper also aids in the formation of bone . . . and works in balance with zinc and Vitamin C to form elastin. . . . One of the early signs of copper deficiency is osteoporosis."[3]

DIABETES AND THE ROLE OF CHROMIUM AND VANADIUM

Diabetes is the third cause of mortality in the West. Its complications are serious and debilitating: blindness, nonfunctioning kidneys that require either dialysis or a kidney transplant, cardiovascular disorders of all kinds that can lead to the necessity of amputations.

In 1957 livestock breeders discovered that diabetes could be both prevented and treated through administering two trace elements: chromium and vanadium. The findings of this research were published in *Federation Proceedings,* the official scientific monthly journal of the National Institutes of Health. According to a study from the University of Vancouver Medical School, vanadium itself can replace the insulin in those suffering from insulin-dependent diabetes (which accounts for 85 percent of all cases of diabetes). Taking a varying dose of vanadium and chromium for a period of four to six months makes it possible to gradually reduce the insulin dose required by the patient until it is no longer needed at all.[4] At the same time it encourages the regeneration of pancreatic tissue that has been damaged by deficiencies of both of these trace elements. It has also been observed that vanadium may protect the body against cancer and cardiovascular diseases.

AGGRESSIVE BEHAVIOR AND LEARNING DISABILITIES AND THE ROLE OF MINERALS

A large number of studies throughout the world have revealed a frequent connection between behavioral problems and certain mineral and vitamin deficiencies. A study at the University of Oregon, for example, demonstrated that the iron found in red blood cells is responsible for carrying large quantities of oxygen to the brain, without which this nerve center cannot function efficiently. Similarly, B Vitamins have been shown to affect the behavior of so-called hyperactive children. The effective synthesis and assimilation of B Vitamins requires the additional minerals calcium and cobalt.

Professor Ruth F. Harrel, a researcher at Old Dominion University in Norfolk, Virginia, led a study to determine whether nutritional deficiencies could be a plausible cause for slow learning and mental retardation and, if so, if it would be possible to treat these conditions with vitamins and minerals. The results were, in her own words, "so extraordinary, that I was scared to believe them." The study continued for eight months and focused on sixteen retarded children whose IQs were somewhere between 17 and 70 (the average IQ is 100). On a daily basis these children were administered nutritional supplements consisting of high doses of eleven vitamins and eight minerals. During the first half of the test period—four months—the IQs of these children improved from 5 to 9.6 points whereas those of the children in the test group receiving placebos showed no change. During the second four-month period the same supplements were also provided to the group that had previously been given placebos, with the result that their IQs improved by at least 10.2 points, a noticeable increase.[5] In fact, all the children in this study benefited significantly from this vitamin/mineral therapy; it was possible to integrate the majority of them into a normal school program after only several months of this treatment.

7
MINERALS:
IN WHAT FORM?

SOME USEFUL DEFINITIONS

Because this book examines minerals, metals, metalloids, trace elements, and colloidal metals, it is important that we have a clear understanding of these and other related terms. This chapter defines these terms and makes clear the distinction between those metals and metalloids found among the hundred or so currently known chemical elements.

Simple body. A simple body cannot be broken down into smaller bodies and consists of only one chemical element. Mandeleev's Table is composed of simple bodies.

Mineral. The dictionary defines a mineral as an inorganic element that is essential to the nutrition of humans, animals, and plants. Minerals are classified as either metals or metalloids. With regard to health and healing, a mineral is an element in the body whose concentration is greater than 1 mg per liter of blood and body fluids.

Metal. A metal is a simple body that is generally a good conductor of heat and electricity and is endowed with a distinguishing shiny surface called a *metallic sheen*. Always solid (with the exception of mercury), metals give off oxides that are most often alkaline. When a nonhydrogenated combination is subjected to electrolysis, the substance that appears in the cathode is always a metal. Furthermore, hydrogenated composites of metals are never acids. The majority of simple bodies are metals, though some—such as bismuth and arsenic—are semimetals, an old name given to substances that are metallic in appearance, brittle, and volatile.

Metalloid. This term refers to any simple body that is nonmetallic.

Trace elements. These are the metalloids or metallic elements that represent only the smallest percentage of the constitutions of living organisms (less than 1 mg per liter of internal fluid). Their presence in trace status, however, is necessary for the growth and life of animals and plants.

Colloidal. This term, meaning "gluelike," is used to describe a system in which the particles of various substances are suspended in fluid as a result of reaching a kind of dynamic equilibrium, which is itself known as a *colloidal state.*

Colloidal Metals and Metalloids (colloidal minerals). These refer to those substances—metals and metalloids—suspended in a state of fine dispersion in a fluid medium. It is possible to obtain such a dispersion of colloidal metals and metalloids by either physical or chemical manipulation—for instance, as Louis De Broglie showed in 1898, by rupturing the electrical arc between two electrodes of the same nonutilizable metal. Here, however, we are interested only in those colloidal metals and metalloids that occur naturally.

Minerals are classified into two broad categories based on their concentration within the cellular environment:

- Mineral salts or minerals whose concentrations are greater than 1 mg per liter
- Trace elements whose concentrations are lower than 1 mg per liter

In current practice, minerals can be presented and prescribed in various basic forms:

As nonorganic minerals. These include oxides, phosphates, carbonates, lactates, sulfates, and so on of calcium, magnesium, zinc, and other minerals. In both the human and the animal body, the bioavailability of nonorganic mineral food supplements is only 8 to 12 percent on average, which falls to 3 to 5 percent among people who are over the age of forty. Nonorganic minerals are the form we most commonly consume, whether we take calcium or zinc tablets or a daily multivitamin/multimineral. Minerals of this kind are generally offered in the form of gluconates (zinc gluconate, calcium gluconate, and so on), carbonates, lactates, sulfates, and oxides. These nonorganic minerals enter the small intestine with essentially a positive charge. If the small intestine's cells also have a net positive charge, the minerals will not be fully absorbed.

As chelated minerals. Particularly valued among the wide array of food supplements, chelated minerals are enclosed within an amino acid, protein, or enzyme. The word *chelation* is derived from the Greek *chele,* which means "claw." A chelated mineral is held as by the "claw" of organized amino acid molecules. In the body, amino acids—the chelating agents in the case of chelated minerals—naturally encircle mineral atoms; isolated metallic atoms do not exist in the body.

Chelation allows a mineral to be more efficient because the body is able to recognize it as a food instead of a foreign body. The body's cells are, in effect, deceived into allowing minerals to enter the body. Minerals that are chelated thus have a bioavailability that is improved by some 25 to 45 percent over that of ingested nonchelated minerals. The most effective form of chelation is that which comes closest to a neutral pH: The positive charge of a mineral becomes neutral or slightly negative, which facilitates the mineral's transport through the intestinal wall to the circulatory system, significantly improving absorption. The most common chelating agents are fumarates, gluconates, picolinates, citrates, and orotates. Most minerals and multiminerals sold in health food stores are chelated. It is important to remember, however, that the reduced bioavailability of nonchelated minerals does not mean that it is useless to take them in this form. We must make the maximum effort to limit mineral deficiencies, even nonchelated supplements produce excellent results. To maximize the benefits of these mineral supplements, they should be taken during meals, so that they can be assimilated at the same time as the rest of our food. They should also be taken over a long period of time; because a large percentage of the supplement's mineral content will be eliminated by the body, thus a daily intake within a long timeframe allows for more absorption.

Certain mineral/vitamin supplements are advertised as "time released." This means they are released gradually into the bloodstream, resulting in an absorption rate can be as much as 40 percent higher than that of formulas that are not time released.

As Schussler salts. Available in either powder or tablet form, these twelve biochemical salts contribute to cells in a form that is a 6/10 dilution of the whole of its constituent elements. Their purpose: to correct any potential mineral deficiencies or excesses.

Through lithotherapy. Here the whole mineral is used, preferably the metal extracted from the mineral. This therapy involves taking minerals (the entire mineral is used or, preferably, the metal extracted from the mineral, in the form of a drinkable homeopathic dilution 8X. Dr. Max Tétau and Dr. Claude Bergeret, originators of this therapy, have selected a range of thirty minerals with determined therapeutic effects in this diluted form.

As Quinton's Marine Plasma and other products that have been developed as part of marine-based therapy. Quinton's Marine Plasma (see chapter 13, page 133), currently available for oral ingestion, encourages cellular regeneration and cellular nutrition, especially through *transmineralization* (penetration of the cell and parts of the internal cellular environment, which is possible due to the small size of the migrating particles). The trace element cocktail it provides is an absolute duplicate of our own internal cellular environment on which it has a balancing effect.

As oligo elements (trace elements). Also known as oligo elements (*oligo* comes from the Greek word meaning "small"), trace elements are mineral substances (both metals and metalloids) present in all living organisms in extremely small, sometimes infinitesimal quantities (hence the name). They represent only about 0.001 percent of body mass—about .25 ounces for a person weighing about 160 pounds! Yet they play an essential biological role and are indispensable to human, animal, and plant life. These can be found commercially under various brand names and are offered in various fluid forms (waters, aqueous extracts, and so forth).

Rare earths are trace elements that we need in even smaller amounts than other trace elements. Among these are lanthanum, praseodymium, neodymium, samarium, europium, ytterbium, yttrium, and thulium.

As colloidal minerals and trace elements. These substances of sea or plant origin can be 98 percent assimilated. They are offered only in liquid form in which the elements themselves exist suspended as very fine particles. Their absorption is 2.5 times greater than that of chelated minerals and 10 times greater than that of nonorganic minerals. Seven thousand times smaller than red blood cells, colloidal minerals are also readily absorbed because they contain a negative charge, while the intestinal wall holds a positive charge. This creates a gradient that concentrates these minerals toward the intestinal mucous, where they are most easily absorbed.

The only place in the world today where it is possible to commercially obtain a mineral cocktail like the one drunk by those long-lived peoples who flourished in high-altitude villages is located in a prehistoric valley of southern Utah. Here nature provides a natural colloidal solution enriched by trace elements accumulated as the water passes through soils dating back some 75 million years. (Indeed, some geologists estimate their age to be 100 million to 150 million years.) While it is possible to obtain colloidal solutions synthetically, it is clear that those offered us by nature directly remain unequalled in quality and provide therapeutic properties that humans and animals have always sought—probably because of the similarity of these solutions to their own internal cellular environment, which is also colloidal by nature. In Part 2, we will examine the vital role of soil in supplying us with the minerals so important to our complete health.

PART 2

Journey to the Center of the Earth: Soils, Springs, and Colloidal Minerals

8

EARTH, SOILS, AND MINERALS

We know that plants take directly from air, water, and earth the elements necessary to sustain life; and that they take these in a mineral form. An animal, however, cannot make use of these same elements unless they have been prepared by plants or by other animals who, either directly or indirectly, have obtained them from plants. It can be stated definitively then that it is the plant that feeds the animal.

LOUIS BERGSON, *CREATIVE EVOLUTION*

We are made to draw our minerals from plants. Yet plants cannot synthesize them if they are not present in the soil. Plants must extract minerals from soil and convert them in their tissues into colloidal minerals, the form in which we store and use the minerals in our own body. Due to the exhausted state of much of the planet's soil, however, our harvests contain but a fraction of what they once held in mineral wealth.

WHAT IS A COLLOIDAL SOLUTION?

A colloidal solution is a stable environment consisting of water and suspended particles. The sole difference between a true solution and a colloidal solution is the number of suspended particles in each. In the case of a true solution, such as one made of sugar and water, particles are small enough to be dispersed evenly throughout the available space. In all living environments, water comes in the form of a colloidal solution, which consists of larger molecules of greater size or larger particles that, despite their size, can be dispersed in water and remain suspended there in a stable balance between the forces of attraction and the forces of repulsion. These submicroscopic particles, called *micells* (from the Latin *mica* meaning "grain" or "particle"), are molecular polymers formed by the combination of some dozen molecules. They retain their identity in suspension, and though their size is supramolecular, which means they are larger than the molecules from which they are formed, they are small enough that a solution containing them remains homogenous. Micell size ranges from a nanometer (10^{-9} m) to 12 micrometers (10^{-5} m), which makes them easily absorbable by the cells of the body.

The molecular structure of micells is characterized by one or more hydrophilic parts (with a strong affinity for water) and one or more lipophilic parts (having a strong affinity for oils, hydrocarbons, and so forth).

Colloidal solutions are common; anyone who has ever made mayonnaise, an emulsified vinaigrette, or whipped cream has created one. Milk is a colloidal solution, as are wine, Chinese ink, and watercolor paints. The most important aspect of a colloidal solution is that it remains stable. A watercolor painting whose colors settle, milk that turns sour, or a mayonnaise that breaks apart has become unstable— a process known as *flocculation.*

How is a stable colloidal solution created? In the case of a solution of oil and water, for example, through the act of shaking or vigorously stirring, the hydrophobic product—oil—is dispersed throughout the solvent—water—in the form of small particles in such a way that the solution maintains homogeneity. A colloidal solution can be thermodynamically stable, which means it will not change over time if the thermodynamic parameters of temperature and pressure do not change. The majority of colloidal solutions, however, are considered *metastable,* meaning that their state will always change after a certain length of time. The stability of these solutions is therefore kinetic.

COLLOIDS IN THE BODY

Living matter is in fact made up of colloids and all body fluids are colloidal solutions.

The suspended state of colloidal solutions is a result of the repulsion of the colloidal particles in the solution due to their like electrical charges. The body's colloidal particles, which carry an electronegative charge, are constantly pushing each other away, thereby maintaining their suspension in the medium.

The phenomenon at play here, then, is electrical in nature. Because of this, we might say that electricity is the bearer of life. Flocculation, or instability, occurs if the electrical balance is upset—for instance, if some enzymatic activity intervenes and causes the colloidal particles to collect in piles. A potential result of this instability is the death of cells and the appearance of organic lesions. According to Dr. Jean-Pierre Willem:

> This organic flocculation appears primarily in infections, organic intoxications (hepatitis, traumas), and even violent emotions. From the aging effects caused by illness, from various assaults against the body or poor hygiene (tobacco, alcohol, stress), we gradually lose our ability to synthesize certain enzymes (formerly known as diastases) and, because of this, the ability to metabolize those substances that our body needs, which accelerates our degeneration.[1]

Colloidal solutions hold an essential place in the organization of living creatures: Cellular fluid, the humoral fluids and blood that bathes the body's tissues, and the sap of trees and plants are all formed in large part from colloidal substances—which highlights the importance of maintaining the "dance of life."

UNBALANCED SYSTEMS: EMULSIONS AND SOILS

Comparing colloidal solutions to emulsions clarifies to some extent the process by which colloidal minerals are conveyed to underground water. In the industrial domain, although it is possible to solubilize large quantities of hydrophobic molecules in aqueous environments with well formulated systems of thermodynamic equilibrium, in the majority of cases it is much more convenient and economical to create metastable, or out-of-balance, systems.

Soils, distinct from emulsions, are the most indispensable metastable systems to all life. In fact, when the ancients spoke of our nourishing world as Mother Earth, we can see that they were not simply speaking metaphorically. Yet few of us are aware of how different substances enter the soil and how this source of trace elements is formed.

An emulsion of oil in water corresponds to the dispersal of one fluid, oil in the form of small droplets, into another fluid, water. Soil, however, consists of small, solid particles dispersed within a fluid medium, most often water.

We must gain a minimal amount of understanding of the constitution of soils and their chemical makeup if we are to have a better understanding of both how plants enrich themselves with minerals during their growth cycles and in turn enrich with minerals and other micellar elements the water passing through them (such as that spring in Utah—see chapter 7 and chapter 12).

This understanding is likewise important because we have reached a time when relations between humans and nature are so strained that the pure and simple survival of the planet—and thus ourselves!—is threatened. Such understanding opens the door to solutions that are urgently needed to restore our world to the healthy state required if we want it to continue to have the capacity to carry us and feed us for much longer.

The most important fact to remember is that soil is a living organism that is far more complex than the most complicated computer. Any intervention in this intricate ecosystem that includes so many organisms results in repercussions that affect the system as a whole and in consequences that cannot always be assessed immediately.

CONSTANT EXCHANGES

First, let us look at how a soil functions and what its physical-chemical properties are.

Among the different constituent elements of soil, the colloids of humus (the relatively stable, organic material of soil) and clay are closely connected and have the capability to exchange both anions (negatively charged ions) and cations (positively charged ions).

This exchange capability along with pH and degree of saturation in metallic cations form the important characteristics of a soil.

Although solid in appearance, soil is in fact a composite solid-fluid mixture that is host to many processes. Constantly altered by the plants that use it as a source of food, the liquid form of soil, known as *soil solution,* contains electrolytes, which, because of their electrical nature, ensure that there is a constant exchange between the liquid and solid forms of the soil. Electrolytes are displaced as an effect of plants' transpiration (the process by which plants take in water from the ground and release it as vapor in the air), and the resulting ionic flux adds to the process of diffusion that brings nutritive elements the plant needs into contact with its roots.

Clay and humus are closely bound to each other, which increases their exchange properties (also known as cation exchange). Because of the variable ionization of organic functions, humus is defined by pH (a 7 pH, on average), which can vary depending on soil quality, the nature and proportion of clays bound to it, and the quantity of organic material it contains. The ability of humus to exchange metallic cations varies with respect to the soil's content of active calcium.

Exchangeable cations can be found in calcium (notably in soils formed from limestone), magnesium, potassium, sodium, and various trace elements (including manganese, copper, and zinc). Iron, which is present in soil in numerous forms, can also play a role in these exchanges.

THE LIQUID PHASE OF SOIL

Generally speaking, the solid constituents of soil are constantly swimming in a liquid phase whose size naturally depends on the state of humidity present. This liquid phase, or soil solution, contains electrolytes—mainly bicarbonates resulting from the decomposition of organic materials by microorganisms. Plants absorb through their roots the nutritive elements from this rich soil solution. The depletion resulting from this absorption is partially compensated for by the release of exchangeable ions or those ions that were present only at the surface of the soil or ground. Also contributing to rebuilding the soil are natural fertilizers such as leaves and the debris of plants and various animals.

These substances dissolve into the soil to add to its reserves. The complex physico-chemistry of soils thus involves the predominant role played by the soil solution through the exchanges of ions among its mineral or organic components.

TRANSFORMATION FROM
ORGANIC MATERIAL TO MINERAL

The organic material found in certain waters, which comes from the decomposition of plants, is a complex blend of polycarbolic acids that are classified as either humic acids or fulvic acids. The concentration of these acids varies according to location of the water and season of the year, with the greatest concentration occurring during the middle of winter.

Residual organic materials from plants and animals—excrement, debris, wastes, corpses—undergo more or less substantial transformations in nature thanks to the activity of microorganisms living in soil and water. The process of turning these materials into compost or humus, which is often rich in barely decomposed debris and which is made up of dark colloidal minerals, is known as *humification*. It also leads to the complete mineralization of organic residues, whether they are fresh or humified beforehand—meaning it transforms these materials into humus.

The transformation of proteins, nitrogen macromolecules in the cells and tissue, into mineral substances is called *ammonification* because the end result of the transformation is ammonia (NH_3). The characteristic odor of this volatile gas is plainly perceptible at certain moments during fermentation when proteins are destroyed.

For many living things, especially chlorophyll-based plant life, nitrogen molecules are assimilated in an ammonia-like form. Incorporated in this form by biological synthesis, they take part in the manufacture of new proteins, which are indispensable in the maintenance of the trophic chain (each level of consumption in the food chain) that leads from plants to animals, who consume and transform organic plant matter.

It is apparent, then, that ammonification is a mandatory link in the cycle that nitrogen follows in nature, whether on the scale of all living things or within a locally formed *biocenosis* (a balanced association of plant and animal life within a certain area).

THE EXCHANGE OF IONS:
A NATURAL PROCESS COPIED BY INDUSTRY

The first scientific observation of ion exchange was made in 1845 by two English chemists, H. S. M. Thompson and J. Spence. While studying the fertilization of soil by ammonium phosphate, they observed that by introducing a solution of this salt into a glass column filled with soil, the ammonia was absorbed and the resulting solution contained calcium sulfate. An exchange had taken place between the calcium cations of the soil and the ammonia cations in the solution.

A similar study was undertaken in 1850 by J. T. Way, who demonstrated the widespread nature of the phenomenon of ion exchange. He also noted that the equal quantities of cations exchanged between the solid and the solution were equivalent and that certain ions were more fixed than others. The first practical application of this research dates from 1905, when R. Gans, in Germany, proved that it was possible to "soften" natural waters—that is, to replace the calcium and magnesium ions they contained with sodium ions by means of natural exchange agents such as those that are aluminocilicate or zeolitic in nature. Soon after, artificial zeolites were created. During the next thirty years zeolites were used worldwide to soften water.

THE ESSENTIAL PROCESS OF AMMONIFICATION

Ammonification involves the decomposition of plant and animal detritus and the transformation of the proteins present in their cells and tissues into mineral substances. Although ammonification in water can be accomplished through photochemical means, it is, overall, a biological process in soil. This is demonstrated by the sensitivity of the process of ammonification to life-limiting factors such as temperature, aeration, and humidity, and by isolating the bacteria responsible for the process. In the ocean there are two ways that organic nitrogen is mineralized via ammonification: In shallow water, bacteria act to produce ammonia and nitrates, but do so rapidly. By contrast, in deep water the process of ammonification is both slower and more intense.

In soil, the medium we are most interested in here, the microflora involved in ammonification operate optimally at a temperature of 30° Celsius and at a soil hydration level of 60 percent of its capacity—both conditions that maintain adequate aeration. These conditions, however, are very infrequently met in those places in nature where ammonification occurs. Yet the microflora responsible for ammonification, taken as a whole, seem to thrive in adverse conditions such as excess alkalinity or acidity; extreme variations in soil temperature, hydration, and humidity; and the absence of adequate air. Such a broad range of tolerances suggests that different kinds of microflora have become relatively specialized, ecologically speaking. Nevertheless, overall, the rate of ammonification owes less to the nature of the microbial population and more to the composition of the organic materials that are actually undergoing the mineralization process, of which ammonification is a part. The rate is slow when the amount of carbon in the decomposing material vastly exceeds the amount of nitrogen, and it is rapid when the opposite is true. This core fluctuation in the rate of ammonification plays a role in seasonal variations of the completed process in both soil and water.

Other factors affecting the rate of ammonification are the texture and structure of the soil itself. The best substratum for ammonification is soil rich in colloidal substances that have been compressed into stable, gritty aggregate. Ammonia formed in this environment is easily affixed to a clay-humus complex. The colloidal spring in Utah happens to be located atop just this kind of substratum.

Finally, beyond the soil itself, worms, insects, mites, and other creatures, with their excrement and excavation, contribute to beneficial structural and microbiological conditions for efficient ammonification and thus a rich mineral content in the soil.

CLAYS AND THEIR COLLOIDAL MINERALS

In large part it is in clay that fields and forests store reserves of plant food. During times of abundance, these miniscule clay particles several thousandths of a millimeter in size are capable of holding water, mineral elements, and certain organic molecules extracted from rain, irrigation, fertilizer, and manure. If conditions of extreme aridity and

THE EARTH IS A LIVING ORGANISM

We should not forget that the earth is a living organism just as complex as our own bodies and those of all other living things. Restricting our understanding of the earth to a purely mechanical and chemical approach would be the equivalent of measuring the internal phenomena of our bodies only through the vantage point of their chemical composition. The hypothesis that the earth is a great, living being has been formulated by, among others, the British scientist James Lovelock in two of his books.* Likewise, ancient traditions maintain that the earth, like us, has a spirit, a soul, and consciousness. This is why shamans from the four corners of the globe consider it with such great respect and deplore the way we treat it today.

This view of the earth also partially explains the marvelous virtues of ancient waters like those in Utah. If their chemical composition has been allowed to enrich itself for millennia without hindrance, we should spare from destruction their energy so that we may reap intact the regenerative powers they offer us.

---

*James Lovelock, *Gaia: A New Look at Life on Earth* (Oxford: Oxford University Press, 1982); and *The Ages of Gaia* (New York: Norton, 1988).

scarcity occur, the clay can then return these stores to plants. In this way, clays serve as a "bank" for plant life.

Oddly enough, clays are the members of the rock family that have most resisted our analysis and understanding because their constituent substances, clayey minerals, are so small they cannot be seen by the naked eye and are difficult to see even with a microscope. Only recently have we discovered their millennia-long history of practical use by humans. In understanding their role it is essential to distinguish the constituent elements—clayey minerals—from their assembling elements—clays mixed with other diverse components. The constituent elements of clays are tiny minerals made up of thin sheets called *leafs* or *lattes* that are measured in thousandths of millimeters, or micrometers. It was only in the twentieth century that mineralogists had the means to identify their structure, nature, and classification.

Clayey minerals generally occur in nature amassed in the form of sheets (hence their name, *phyllites,* from the Greek *phyllon,* meaning "leaf") and, like mica, they belong to the family of phyllosilicates. Each crystal of phyllite is composed of several hundred stacked layers that are measured in nanometers a thousand times smaller than micrometers. The structure of the first layer distinguishes this type of mineral from other types.

It is easy to see how carefully, on the scale of a millionth of a millimeter, crystalline structure is formed. Out of these variations come the different types of clayey minerals:

- Kaolinite combines a tetrahedron-shaped layer of silicium and an octahedron-shaped layer of aluminum.
- Illites combine, like mica, an octahedron-shaped layer that is mostly aluminum with two tetrahedron-shaped layers composed primarily of silica.
- Smectites form a large group built on the same model as the illites, but the stacking of each of the elementary sheets is irregular in relation to the plane of the previous sheet.
- Chlorites are constructed similarly to illites, smectites, and micas, but the interfoliated space between chlorites' layers is taken up by a contiguous layer of various kinds of hydroxides.
- Interstratified clayey minerals are minerals that consist of alternating sheets or, most often, different interfoliated spaces. Interstratified minerals represent the transformational stage of one clayey mineral into another.
- Minerals made up of plates (broader and thicker than a leaf), sepiolites and attapulgites are composed not only of stacked sheets, but also of three-layer bands.

Clayey Rocks

Clayey rocks are a blend of clayey minerals and various other minerals present in nature and include, among others, sandy clays, limestone or marl clays, bituminous clays. For a rock to be considered a clay it is necessary that the proportion of clayey minerals be large enough to imbue the material as a whole with its attributes such as thinness, fragility, and plasticity, as well as properties such as its well-known ability of absorption.

Clays and clayey rocks are not found in the zones deep in the earth's crust. They are silicates that are instead found in the three zones closest to the surface of the earth: the zone affected by changes in meteorological conditions, the zone comprising lakeside or marine sedimentation, and the zone where *diagenesis* (all the physical, chemical, and biological changes that affect sediment after it is initially deposited) occurs through burial and where hydrothermal activity (such as the spring in Utah) occurs.

The Birth of Clays

Any of three different mechanisms may be operative in the formation of clays or clayey minerals:

- Neoformation, in which clayey minerals are created on site through the combination of ions present in solutions. These minerals are characteristic of the places that created them.
- Inherited formation, which is the opposite of neoformation. In this process, minerals have been introduced from elsewhere and have accumulated at a particular place. They may date from the past and have remained intact within the rock, much like the property we inherit from our ancestors. For this reason, inherited minerals characterize the ancient or remote sites where they were created, but not the area where they are found.
- Transformation, which is characterized by minerals that have resulted from inherited formation but have evolved to take on new status as a result of their new environment. A distinction is made between transformation that results from degradation, meaning that something has been taken away from the substance, and those that result from the intake of new ions that have combined with the substance. Minerals may also be transformed through recrystallization. The status of minerals formed in this way is regarded as intermediary, as their substance is inherited but their structure has been newly created. Through these intermediary minerals nature transitions from one of the three mechanisms of formation and another.

Clays from the Weathering Zone

Rocks of all kinds on the planet's surface are exposed to meteorological activity such as rain, snow, cold, and heat, as well as conditions of humidity and aridity. Rock changes as a result of the effects of all of these and is quickly colonized by living organisms such as plants, animals, and bacteria.

Weathering conditions and soils on the planet's surface vary according to climatic zones. Because of this, around the world vast areas exist in which soil and alterations reveal either one of the three mechanisms of clay formation or complete dissolution. These clays are recognizable because, when broken down into sediment, the climatic conditions of their origins can be reconstructed.

Clays Resulting from Inherited Formation

The clays inherited from the continental masses have lent themselves to the formation of lakes created by rivers, glacial lakes, and the ocean floors from the shores of the continents to the border of the great oceanic depths. Rivers and streams deliver additional clays inherited from mother rocks and soils and ground cover affected by weather. Demonstration of this can be shown by two extreme examples. In the *flyschs* and *molasses* (strata occurring primarily in the mountains), clays came directly from still living cordilleras or steep sided mountain chains; here illites and chlorites are the predominant minerals. At the opposite extreme, we have the siderolitic facies in which kaolinite and iron oxides from a continental layer of lateritic soils are accumulated.

Today's oceans illustrate the influence of the climate zones that rule over the continents. At the equator the rivers carry predominantly kaolinite, while smectites come from every region. The temperate zones are the realm of degraded and interstratified minerals whose core variations allow us to reconstruct the climatic variations of the Quaternary period. Finally, illites and chlorites from mother rocks come from glacial platforms and living cordilleras. We should note that this organized system can be disturbed by underwater currents and the arrival of altered smectites in volcanic ash.

Transformation

The greater the difference between a newer sedimentary environment or microenvironment and a mineral's original environment, the more dramatic the transformation. Research has demonstrated the gradual transformation of clays inherited into magnesium smectites in Lake Chad in Africa. In general, in the epicontinental lake beds created on the cusp of the Cretacean/Eocene eras, as well as in many tertiary lake beds, there is evidence of the gradual transformation, followed by recrystallization, of aluminum smectites, magnesium smectites, and even attapulgites.

Neoformations

As the neoformations of sepiolite, hectorite, and stevensite in lakeside basins (such as those of Ghazul in Morocco and Sommières in France) indicate, minerals can be born directly out of the ions in a solution state. The concentration of ions in these instances is a result of evaporation. But other clayey minerals are created in an oceanic environment. For example, the glauconites, a kind of ferriferous illites, are created through neoformation or recrystallization. The neoformations that appear in the great ocean depths are quite spectacular. The red clays from these areas, which include newly formed ferriferous smectites (such as zeolites) now cover a quarter of the globe. These new minerals are the products of dissolving limestone silt, silica silt, and volcanic ash. These metamorphoses in the depths of the world's oceans are the counterpart of the weathering changes that affect the continental land masses.

THE THERAPEUTIC PROPERTIES OF CLAYS

Understanding the complex properties of clays[3] makes it possible to better grasp their individual therapeutic virtues and thus use them to greater effect. While it remains true that simple green clay (generally of Montmorillonite origin) is often perfectly suitable for achieving desired therapeutic results, the genesis and mineral composition of other varieties of clay demonstrate the range of therapeutic values that we could expect them to deliver—though these varieties may be difficult to find.

It is easy to see why ancient peoples who had the good fortune to know of unexploited and remote deposits of a variety of natural clays considered these places to be sacred sites that possessed magical powers.

A Very Long History

Clay has a long and venerable history that reaches back millennia. In the book of Genesis, for instance, God molds Adam from clay. In their creation stories, some Amerindians are even more specific, offering that white clay was used for this task.

Egyptian papyri reveal that as early as 3000 B.C. the physicians who attended the pharaoh made wide use of yellow ochre—a clayey earth containing iron oxide—to treat all manner of illnesses, wounds, skin lesions, and inflammations, and that embalmers used clay blended with essential oils in the mummification of the dead.

Ancient Greeks called their clay Lemnos earth after the island on which it was found and quarried. The Greek physician Galen (129 –212? A.D.), a philosopher of ancient Greece and Rome and the father of modern medicine, went to this island to study the effects of the clay on dysentery, intoxication, hemorrhaging, digestive troubles, and even the plague.

In his *Natural History,* Pliny the Elder mentions the virtues of a kind of white earth that could be found in the vicinity of Naples. When cleaned, dried, and reduced to a powder, this earth had the reputation of protecting from numerous ailments. The Gospels also refer to the therapeutic use of clay, telling us that Jesus restored sight to a blind man by making a paste of clay and applying it to the eyes of the afflicted individual.

As we can see, there is a wealth of stories from all times and from every continent that boast the virtues of this miraculous earth. The Arab doctor Avicenna, Marco Polo, Mahatma Gandhi, and many others have advised its use, and some ancient peoples even ingested it. Among the Dogons of what are present-day Mali and its neighboring countries, it was so revered that those who worked with it to make pottery were considered to possess magic powers. In the Himalayas, some Tibetan peoples took red clay to prevent goiter. From Sudan to the Middle East, from Mexico and India to the Mississippi Delta, clay was considered a sovereign remedy against countless maladies.

In using clay therapeutically, humans were probably duplicating the behavior of the animals around them who have always turned to clay-rich mud as a remedy for their ills.

The mineral richness of clay comes in large part from the plant world. Because clay serves as a kind of "bank" for plant life, it can cleanse and purify the human body, enrich the blood of those who are anemic by increasing iron levels, heal skin disorders, and fill the body's mineral deficiencies.

Clay's efficacy in correcting these deficiencies is due to its richness in natural colloidal minerals of plant origin. The elements in clay act as catalysts whose presence makes it possible for the body to affix and incorporate those substances that it has been unable to retain. Best of all, only a small quantity of clays are required for therapeutic results: Usually only one tablespoon per day can achieve the desired results.

SEVERAL CLAYS USED THERAPEUTICALLY

If you are fortunate enough to have access to a variety of clay deposits, however they might be, the following summaries should help you to assess them and determine their most likely therapeutic applications. Of course, this is only a partial list, a sampling of the earth's many regenerative clays.

So-called Green Clay

It should be noted that there is a wide variety of green clays whose qualities—and virtues—vary significantly. The best of these is Montmorillonite (which actually might be green, white, or even blue). Very rich in magnesium, this clay contains silica, iron oxide, aluminum, manganese oxide, lime, magnesium oxide, potassium, soda, titanium oxide, and phosphates. Its absorption capacities as well as its purity make it far superior to other green clays.

It is detoxifying, remineralizing, and absorbent. This is the clay most commonly used in a variety of applications because of its diverse properties. It is used either externally in the form of a poultice or is taken internally, diluted in water, to restore minerals and to purge the body of toxins and other impurities. In cases of anemia, one glass daily of "clay milk" (one tablespoon of green clay dissolved in a glass of water) can help to increase the red blood cell count.

White Clay or Kaolinite

The first known deposit of this clay in Kao Ling, China, gives it its name, but it can also be found in France (Brittany and Limoges) and England. Created from the decomposition of granite, it consists of two layers, silica and aluminum

In the form of clay milk, it has strong coating action as well as anti-bacterial, anti-inflammatory, and healing properties that make it preferable to other clays as protection and healing promoter for the gastric and intestinal mucous membrane. In addition, it halts fermentations and absorbs toxins, making it valuable in instances of bloating or food poisoning. It also acts as bulk, which helps in the fight against constipation and helps to regulate pH. All external treatments are indicated: poultices, plasters, and packs. It is excellent as a mouthwash and as a baby powder.

German Green Clay or Ludos

This clay, either beige or grayish-orange in color, is the most popular in use in Germany. It shares all the same qualities as Montmorillonite.

Attapulgite

White, green, and sometimes bright red, its strong absorption properties lead to its therapeutic use in gastric dressings and to treat stomach ulcers, colitis, and gastritis. Attapulgite is also used in the manufacture of cat litter.

Illite

Widespread in northern France, this common clay, which has a high calcium content and is quite low in magnesium, will adhere tightly to the skin when applied. Its strong absorption properties make it especially useful in absorbing wastes and impurities. When applied as a thick poultice, it reduces swelling in sprains, twisted wrists and ankles, and the like.

Bentonite

Its name comes from Fort Benton in the state of Montana, where a large deposit of this clay is located. It provides a good base for medications and cosmetics because it encourages the skin's absorption of their elements.

Octalite
This is particularly recommended in cases where waste remains too long in the digestive tract and begins to ferment.

Diosmectite
This mineral is used in the treatment of digestive disorders, including infant diarrhea.

HUMUS AND ITS COLLOIDAL MINERALS

Humus, you will recall is arable earth, a blackish colloidal substance that is the result of the partial decomposition of plant and animal wastes. It is that beautiful black dirt in which most plants delight and prosper and, in doing so, generate our own health and vitality.

The colloids in humus are hydrophilic, meaning they are thirsty for water, which when present causes them to swell. If, however, they are subjected to a prolonged arid period, they can become hydrophobic and only gradually become rehydrated

These hydrophilic colloids are negative ions and their negative charges allow them to play an important role in the soil's ability to absorb cations. The "exchange capacity" of humic colloids—in other words, the maximum amount of cations they are capable of absorbing—is higher than that of clay, somewhere on the order of 2 to 5 milliequivalents* per gram.

RECYCLING OR HOW SOIL ENRICHES ITSELF

In every ecosystem on earth, the elements necessary for life (biogenetic elements) are successively incorporated into different living compounds (plants, animals, microflora), through which they are then released. It could be said that there is a renewal or "turnover" (as another term for recycling) of these elements. This cyclical transformation of elements is as indispensable to the maintainance of life on earth as is the solar energy that is constantly being harnessed by photosynthetic organisms.

---

*A milliequivalent is the scientific unit for something so small that it defies measurement.

Plant remains and microbial cells are incorporated into the soil with animal remains, where they form a complex of organic matter that has not yet been transformed into humus. One part of this complex is subsequently mineralized and reabsorbed by plants and another part is humified. The residual compounds constituting humified organic matter then gradually combine with the mineral particles of the soil to form the organoclay compartment that plays a major role in those soils whose clay content is higher than 10 percent.

All mineral elements contained in soil can be rendered in solution form by microorganisms, chiefly bacteria, which allows us to avoid resorting to chemical fertilizers. As we might presume, this mineralization of organic matter occurs all the more rapidly when the organic matter itself decays rapidly. In this way, mineralization of organic phosphorus occurs in parallel to the process of ammonification.

A SITE OF INTENSE LIFE

Far from being inert matter, the earth is animated by life that, in its variety and ceaseless activity, renders our planet extraordinary. An important contingent of the earth's life are those organisms that assist in the breakdown of plants into humus and, ultimately, nourishment for plants and humans.

The work of scholars such as Schloesing, Laurent, and Truffaut has shown that, beyond manure or animal excrement, soil has two other sources for the carbohydrates necessary to synthesize humus.

1. The radical breakdown of plants that exude sugars—carbohydrates—which bacteria take in exchange for their nitrogen.
2. Microscopic algae living on the soil's surface, in the light and in the top millimeters of the arable layer. These are essentially miniature plants that, thanks to their chlorophyll, can synthesize carbohydrates, which leads to the transformation of minerals into organic matter.

Encouraging the proliferation of these algae also encourages that of nitrifying bacteria, and therefore the enrichment of the soil with nitrogen and soluble minerals that enable plants to eat. Unfortunately, it just so happens that current conventional farming methods encourage the exact opposite.

In our choice of farming practices, it is important to remember that soil is a living environment that is much more sensitive and fragile than is generally believed. It is necessary, for instance, to avoid at all costs overwhelming or disturbing its biological activity by working the soil in a way that is counterproductive or that overwhelms its structure.

The fact is that microorganisms and all the tiny life forms inhabiting soil play a predominant role in the nutrition and growth of plants. They are the principal agents of the decay of the soil's organic matter, which they transform into mineral or organic substances that plants can assimilate. As Claude Aubert puts it, "Experience shows that only those soils that are rich in humus and endowed with an intense biological activity are capable of producing healthy and vigorous plants."[4]

The flora and fauna inhabiting our soil include countless invisible species, such as protozoa, nematodes, enchytraeidae, tardigrades, mites, springtails, fungi, bacteria, algae, and so forth, not to mention the common earthworm. The preservation of all these living beings is essential to the life of the soil—including what plants it grows and how it grows them. The mechanical and biochemical roles of such organisms is far from negligible. It follows from this that certain farming methods that pay no heed to the survival of these sometimes unseen creatures contributes to the sterilization of our soils. Extensive tilling of the earth, for instance, buries those organisms that can live only on or near the surface of the soil and brings to the surface those that are unable to tolerate it. In addition, among the wide variety of chemical products available to farmers are those that are extremely harsh on all life forms.

THE BIOCHEMICAL ACTIVITY OF EARTHWORMS

These friendly little animals deserve a far better fate than ending up at the end of a fishing line or left in a pitiable state on our sidewalks and roads. The activity they provide that is essential to the enrichment of our soil should compel not only our attention but also protective measures and respect.

The tunnels they dig aerate the soil, making it more permeable to the penetration of air and water, but their digging activity also blends together the soil's various constituent elements, pushing back to the surface some from deep in the ground and bringing to deeper areas those from the surface. Earthworms also absorb plant wastes, which they eventually expel in the form of excrement after having reduced them to fine particles blended with dirt.

Studies cited by Claude Aubert have shown that in comparison to the surrounding soil, the excrement of earthworms is:

- Five times richer in nitrogen in the form of nitrates
- Two times richer in exchangeable calcium
- Two and one half times richer in exchangeable magnesium
- Seven times richer in absorbable phosphorus
- Eleven times richer in exchangeable potassium.

It seems earthworms can achieve the same phenomenon with trace elements: In New Zealand it was shown that it was possible to eliminate molybdenum deficiencies (in soils that were rich in this substance but not in absorbable molybdenum) by a simple addition of earthworms to the soil. It is also known that tilling prairie soils sometimes leads to deficiency-based diseases. Interesting, it so happens that such tilling is always followed by a sharp drop in the earthworm population.[5]

It has been estimated that an earthworm absorbs its own weight in soil every day, which would amount to some 300 grams a year, and that the weight of the dirt transported by earthworms in an old prairie environment that is still full of life runs close to 60 tons per year.

FARMING THAT RESPECTS THE SOIL

We have seen how soil ideally should contain all the elements plants need, and in the form and proportions that are most usable to them. Based on the research of Liebig, it has been accepted that plants essentially absorb organic substances and their food in the form of mineral ions present in the soil.

Nitrogen fertilizers often used in agriculture cause an accelerated mineralization of the soil's organic reserves, thus a net loss of humus and a reduction in the soil's fertility.

Every gardener, even an amateur one, can see that not all plants like the same kind of soil. Some plants prefer soils that are more acid, others prefer soils that are more alkaline or even neutral. Some plants prefer loose soil, whereas others do best in thick clays. The same diversity is at play in climate preferences. It is obvious that respecting the preferences of the plants we wish to grow should be one of the basic rules of thumb for a sane and logical farming system. Yet such consideration is far from the case in commercial agriculture today, where economic imperatives trump natural laws. The laws of economics provide yet another reason to "force" plant growth with the help of toxic chemicals.

There are certain basic rules for an agricultural practice that respects the soil and the natural life cycles that take place there, leading to the production of healthy, high quality plants. Two of these rules involve:

- The principle of crop and soil rotation, which allows the land the time it needs to regenerate
- The avoidance of tilling and plowing, which destroys the soil's surface, arable layer and the coherence of the different layers beneath this first layer and disrupts the microflora and microfauna present throughout the soil. If all the bacteria and other anaerobic life of the soil's deeper layers are suddenly deposited on its surface, while all those that thrive on the surface are buried, the soil simply "dies."

The Jean Method,[6] often applied in agro-biology, provides a viable alternative. Among other things, it advocates replacing plowing with superficial "scrapings" that are intended to aerate the soil and help it to retain its humidity. Each scraping gradually increases the arable layer by 3 to 6 cm, depending on the nature of the soil and how dry it is. In addition, any grass or weed growth is destroyed each time the cultivator is passed over the plot (generally every fifteen days).

PLANTS AND THEIR MINERALS

Helpful to our understanding of the endless cycle of depletion and renewal of soil is a basic understanding of the way plants absorb nutrients and establish the syntheses within that are key to their survival—and our own.

The Absorbent Hairs

The great majority of plants draw from the soil the water and mineral salts they need. These minerals of course come to them in their natural colloidal form, and plants essentially draw their nourishment from these nutritive microcells. The tiny hairs on the plant's young roots play an essential role by absorbing in ion state the mineral elements in the liquid phase of soil, whether directly from this soil solution or from colloids on the ground to which they have been fixed by adsorption. These ions can be freed or introduced into organic complexes that support them.

Absorption is affected by a number of factors some of which are connected to the plant and others to the environment. Both aeration and temperature are influential, as is the physiological state of the plant's tissues and the implementation of metabolic processes. The mechanisms at play in this absorption are essentially the same as those occurring in intercellular transport: osmosis in the case of water and, in the case of ions, passive diffusion and the membranous enzymatic pumps of influx and efflux.

For plants that grow in the ground, the absorption of water and mineral elements is essentially performed by the roots' absorbent hairs, highly elongated giant cells that are located near the tips of the roots. They have considerable density (up to 2500 per cm^2 among the graminaceous plants, which include grasses, bamboo, and sugar cane). It has been estimated that a square foot of rye has roots that equal 250 km in length, translating to an absorbent surface of 470 m^2. Contributing to the absorbing capability of each of the root hairs are its vast surface area (which multiplies by a factor of 2 to 10 times that of the roots), thin membrane, and large vacuole. Absorbent hairs are rare among trees (including oak and beech), and are absent from many conifers such as pine. Aquatic plants, except for those that live in total darkness, have no absorbent hairs, and algae, for their part, absorb through their entire surface area.

The soil volume available to the plant is even larger given the fact that the liquid phase of the soil forms a relatively coherent fluid network. A plant is capable of attracting the ground water and salts it finds dissolved several centimeters and even several decimeters away.

Atmospheric water—either fog or dew—can be absorbed by the aerial roots (those that run along the surface of the ground). Such is the case in desert environments, where there is a particular abundance of nocturnal dew. Leaves also help with the absorption of water in natural conditions. Through measurement, we have been able to determine that the values of plant water intake are quite high; roughly stated, a plant daily absorbs at least its own weight in water. The mass of mineral elements absorbed is far less because these must cover only the plant's nutritive requirements. Properly speaking, a plant absorbs ions rather than elements. In the case of potassium, for example, it is not the metal K that is at work in the nutrition of the plant but the cation K+.

PHYTOTHERAPY AND THE NUTRITIONAL PROPERTIES OF PLANTS

While the aromatic properties of plants are most often given the greatest consideration in phytotherapy, we must also acknowledge the other properties and constituents that plants contribute. Among these are vitamins, enzymes, minerals, and trace elements. It is more than likely that a large portion of the virtues of medicinal plants is due to their mineral content. Chamomile, for example, contains 1800 mg of potassium per 200 calories. In addition, 23 percent of its makeup is calcium. The dry extracts of some cactus varieties consist of 80 percent calcium. Horsetail contains a high amount of silicic acid.

Naturally, the medicinal plants having a high mineral content are generally reputed to heal disorders related to mineral deficiencies. It is easy to see that nature planned for us to maintain a certain balance of minerals and trace elements in our body through the consumption of certain plants. We can choose which vegetables to eat based on their richness in the elements that are necessary for our health.

While we can't list here the mineral constituents of all common vegetables, it is interesting to note that garlic, for example, is an excellent source of sulfur, iodine, silica, and selenium, and that carrots, which are a good source of carotene, are also full of calcium, sodium, potassium and—especially in its leaves—magnesium. Cabbage provides iron, copper, magnesium, iodine, and traces of arsenic (which is non-toxic in its natural form). More information on the mineral and trace element content of various vegetables and plants is readily available in herbals and other books related to phytotherapy.

As this chapter on soils and how plants extract nutrients from them has shown, our important task is to preserve the mineral content of our soil and enable, rather than inhibit, the natural cycles that replenish it.

ORIGINS OF SOILS AND CLAYS

Paleosols or Fossil Soils

Paleosols and fossil soils are ancient soils that are extremely rich in minerals and trace elements of all kinds. It is through these almost miraculously preserved pockets of ancient earth that the Utah spring flows, rich in colloidal trace elements.

Among the numerous factors contributing to soil formation—mother rock, climate, relief, animal and plant organisms, weather—it is climate that plays the main role. During the Quaternary period alone, a wide variety of climatic events took place across the planet, resulting in dramatic changes in the process of the formation and evolution of the earth's soil. Because pedologists are often hard pressed to explain the genesis of certain soils under current climate conditions, they look to the significance of ancient conditions that presided over the birth of such soils, which they term paleosols or fossil soils. We should note that most often paleosols are covered by more recent formations, as is the case with the site of the spring in Utah, or have been buried through many cycles of erosion and deposit.

Soils that have developed more recently have been subject to only a single climatic phase and show characteristics related to the conditions they experience at present. These soils have developed naturally, but their occurrence is rare. There are also soils that are covered by a variety of deposits, including alluvial deposits, eolian deposits, and volcanic deposits. Most of the earth's soils, however, are old and have undergone a series of changes from climatic conditions that are quite different from those that exist around them today.

The Clays Resulting from Decalcification

When rainwater charged with carbon gas dissolves limestone and dolomites, the resulting insoluble residues are mainly clays, from silica and iron oxide, that equal as much as 10 percent of the original rock. These insoluble residues of carbonate rock, known as the clays of decalcification, have most often been transported from their original site or modified and mixed with alluvial, eolian, or colluvial substances to create what is known as terra calcis, which include the terra fusca and terra rossa.

Terra fuscas contain hydrated iron oxides that impart an ochre tint. These soils were formed in the hot, moist climate of an interglacial period followed by a cold period that ensured the addition of limestone fragments to the mix. Today terra fuscas are found in temperate climate zones as brown calcic or calcimagnesic soils and leached brown soils.

Terras rossas are characterized by their red color, which is due to the dehydration of iron salts. They were initially formed in a hot and humid climate alternating with extremely dry seasons that would have encouraged this dehydration process. These soils, formed during interglacial periods, are 50,000 or 60,000 years old at the least, and probably much older. Currently they function as mother rock that gives birth to different kinds of soils depending on local climate conditions.

Siderolithic Soils

In 1909 E. Fleury defined siderolithic formation:

> Under the name siderolithic is included an entire geological formation that is very complex and specialized, that is infinitely variable in appearance, and ordinarily characterized by iron minerals in grains or pisoliths, which represent only a relatively small portion of the deposit. They are in fact always closely bound, combined, or subordinated to ferruginous clays, silici sands, and even limestone.

Siderolithic formations have been recognized in three eras—the Carboniferous, Lower Cretacean, and Eocene—and at high latitudes (such as, in France, the edges of the Central Massif, Poitou, Vendée, Charente, the Parisian basin, Boulannais, and the regions of Bray and those of the Upper Marne). They were formed in humid, tropical conditions. Following the transformations that occurred at the end of the Tertiary Period, siderolithic formations were likely partially exhumed during the Quaternary Period, making it a polycyclic fossil soil. In the zones where it has been exhumed, it behaves like mother rock on which primarily leached soils and podzolic soils develop.

Flint Clay

The term *flint clay* designates formations of variable structure and constitution whose commonality is that they contain silex existing in a crumbly matrix that can be clay, clay and sand, or even more rarely, sand or silt. Silex clays are rich in kaolinite and iron oxides. Their density is variable but is rarely more then ninety feet. They seem to have emerged in large part from the metamorphosis of chalk-white formations of flint. Their formation would have been particularly intense in the era during which Nummulitic fossils were formed under the influence of a hot, humid climate, whereas other flint clays, differentiated by their mineralogical make-up, would have been formed during the Neocene era. After their formation, silex clays were likely covered over by sand or silt and sometimes would have combined with these materials.

Certain flint clays exist atop tertiary formations of primarily the Miocene and Oligocene epochs and can therefore be considered as buried fossil soils. When running water, such as springs or underground rivers, passes through these old soils trace elements that have accumulated for thousands or even hundreds of thousands of years leach from the earth, enriching the water in many ways.

In the next chapter we shall turn from soil to water, looking more closely at this substance so necessary to life.

9
WATER: THE
SOURCE OF LIFE

It is premature to seek to reduce the vital processes to the
clearly insufficient concepts of 19th-century or even 20th-
century physico-chemistry.

LOUIS DE BROGLIE

The symbol of abundance and fertility, water has played a fundamental
role in the birth and development of life on this planet. Indispensable to
the formation and nutrition of all living things, it in fact permeates our
entire body. Water, neither passive nor neutral, is far from having dis-
closed all its secrets.

Every civilization for as far back as we can remember has wor-
shiped sacred springs and fountains and attributed to them magical
properties. The large majority of sites used in Christian worship, for
example—from the great cathedrals to the thousands of tiny chapels
lost in the wild and dedicated to various saints—were built atop sacred
springs that were worshipped by the Celts. Because they continued to
enjoy a reputation for unique properties as Christianity became a dominant force, these "powers" were subsequently explained as having
come from a saint or saints who lived at or spent time at the site of the
miraculous water. For instance, the water from the sacred spring at

Lourdes is still venerated and continues to provide healing. And there are many more such sites, obscure, hidden on mountainsides, whose forgotten virtues have left no trace except perhaps the ruins of an ancient hermitage dedicated to an unknown saint.

The Indians of America also worshipped springs where they believed nature spirits dwelled—spirits that guided them and taught them how to cure their fellow humans as well as animals. The Hupas and Yuroks of Northern California as well the Lakota, Iroquois, and other nations all knew water chants that had been transmitted to them by these spirit beings who were endowed with healing powers.

These natural springs do in fact have healing properties, due to being enriched by passing through ancient, uncultivated soil that has not been exhausted of its mineral content. Such waters provided (and sometimes still provide) a solution rich in micells and colloidal minerals that confer upon them their particular therapeutic properties.

WATER: AN ENERGY HARNESSER

Water, the most abundant substance on the surface of the planet, exists in three different material states. Best-known in the form of snow and ice, water in a solid state is also present in countless minerals—the natural hydrates. In their liquid state, natural waters are blends in which hydrogen oxide mixes with mineral or organic impurities. Water in its vaporous state is an important constituent of the earth's atmosphere.

Although the subject of much study, most of the physicochemical properties of water are still poorly known. A liquid with recognized uncommon thermodynamic properties, however, it is water that even today serves as the reference element in the Celsius thermometric scale.

A chemical compound of oxygen and hydrogen, water is the famous H_2O discovered by Lavoisier and Gay-Lussac more than three centuries ago. It consists of three atoms: one of oxygen and two of hydrogen. Its two opposing electrical poles (the hydrogen atom, $H+$, is a positive proton whereas its $OH-$ counterpart is negative) are the cause of its incessant molecular activity, making it quite different from the stable, inert mass that some scientists once believed it to be. In addition, water upends many scientific rules. For example, any other compound that solidifies under the effect of cold becomes more dense and sinks to the bottom of a container—but ice floats. In fact, in its liquid state, water possesses a very unique molecular organization: The two hydrogen atoms are arranged on either side of the oxygen atom but form an angle of about 105 degrees—slightly more open than a right angle. It is this distinctive arrangement that confers upon the water molecule its odd electrical properties. As we have seen, oxygen is electronegative while hydrogen is electropositive—which gives the water molecule an oxygen pole with a negative tendency opposed to a hydrogen pole that is positive. This makes it sensitive to the electrostatic attractions coming from neighboring water molecules as well as to any body holding an electrical charge.

The water molecule, when it is broken apart—as is the case in an electrolyte solution—divides into two unequal parts: H on one side, OH on the other. This inequality generates the appearance of an electromagnetic oscillation of a very high frequency, which led Louis-Claude Vincent to state, "Water creates life non-stop because it is a heterodyne multi-vibrator capable of vitalizing inert matter with the aid of all the vibrations it receives from the universe." In physics a receiver capable of changing the frequency of the waves it receives is labeled *heterodyne*. Energy is required to maintain this oscillating activity. Electromagnetic rays with which water can resonate, particularly those generated by solar radiation, provide this energy. This is why water that is fabricated synthetically, and is toxic by nature, can lose this toxicity by being exposed for several days to sunlight which makes it "biological"—which is to say, capable of playing its intended role inside a living organism.

It is clear to see that water is in no way an inert solvent as it was once thought to be. In nature there is no such thing as pure water; it always contains different bodies either in solution or in suspension.

Marcel Violet, An Unjustly Ignored Researcher

Marcel Violet's experiments made it possible to provide evidence of the radiation that is capable of transforming the biological properties of water. For this purpose he subjected water samples to electromagnetic waves from the entire range of all known frequencies. He began getting results when he started using a special oscillator equipped with condensers whose dielectric (an insulating and nonconducting material) was made from beeswax. This apparatus, known as the Violet Oscillator, made it possible to restore water's remarkable biological properties in several hours. Experiments performed by Etienne Guillé have shown that water treated by the Violet Oscillator has a very revitalizing effect on plants and animals, including humans.

Electrodes fashioned from various metals were subsequently created for use with this oscillator. These made it possible to generate vitalized colloidal solutions rich in trace elements.

Louis-Claude Vincent

The founder of bioelectronics, Louis-Claude Vincent, a hydrological engineer, believed that only his method made it possible to understand organic functioning, how illnesses appeared and developed, and the effect of treatment. It was his belief that it was necessary to measure three values in order to comprehend the properties of an aqueous solution: its pH, its rH2 (or redox potential) and its resistivity.

These three factors have a universal scope and condition all vital activities, from plant growth to the development of microorganisms, from the fertility to overall health of animals and humans. Too little used today, bioelectronics has a large field of potential applications that should make it part of the essential foundation for the medicine of the future. It is a technique too complex to be summed up here, yet it must be emphasized that Vincent's research has allowed us to spectacularly advance our understanding of water's mysteries. For example, in 1950 in Lebanon, he observed that bacteria proliferate in a reductive environment whereas, conversely, disinfection by oxidizing agents such as chloride, encourages the propagation of viruses. Data like this, though generally overlooked, could open a good many doors in the field of medicine.

André Simoneton

André Simoneton, another engineer, established a scale of known waves that made it possible for him to determine which waves possessed favorable or unfavorable factors for health. According to Simoneton, the human body emits waves in the neighborhood of 6200/7000 angstroms, a rate that is necessary to maintain good health. Again according to Simoneton, our entire environment plays a role in our "radiation," which he also called *biovitality* and which consists of the bath of waves in which we live (such as cosmic and telluric waves) and the waves of the foods we eat and the water we drink and in which we bathe.

In his study of water he asserted that when it is too pure—as is the case with distilled water—it is lifeless and so will subtract some of the body's vitality to restore its own balance. Further, "All water is vitalized by contact with a mineral . . . or anything that projects waves . . . and retains for a certain period the radiations it has received."[1] It would be this contact with minerals that allows water to carry waves. Simoneton believed that people should drink only vitalized water. Among these he included seawater, mountain water—particularly that from glaciers (glacier's milk) and certain deep springs.

Simoneton suggested that there are various procedures that can serve to revitalize water that is no longer naturally vital, one of which would be the addition of metallic ions, to wit trace elements or minerals. Results can also be obtained with the simple addition of several drops of lemon or orange juice—all it takes to create a colloidal mineral solution! Water that has been vitalized in this way is easily digested, light, pleasant-tasting, and favorable to health. Thermal waters are especially effective with this addition because of their elevated radiation levels from their mineral activity. Thermal waters imbibed straight from their source are especially vitalized. This is why it is necessary to drink only small portions of them at a time in order to avoid prompting too strong a "reaction." When bottled, such waters exhibit rapid reduction of their radiation, and after about two weeks there is little left of their initial radiation.

We must note one seemingly odd conclusion of Simoneton: Having analyzed water taken from the famous grotto at Lourdes, he believed that it would cure only when used for bathing. He concluded that the explanation for the miracles attributed to it essentially stemmed from its very high level of radiation (15,600 angstroms), connected to the presence of mineral ions. This would also account for the fact that although many people suffering from contagious diseases have bathed regularly in these pools, "there has never been . . . any contagion passed on because of the high energy of this water." If this is the case, perhaps it is also true of Italy's San Damiano spring, whose radiation, at 14,000 angstroms, is almost equal to that of the waters at Lourdes.

THE MIRACLES OF LOURDES: ONE HYPOTHESIS

According to André Simoneton:

> It is because doctors do not (or cannot) yet calculate the beneficial value of the ions in mineral waters through the precise calibration of their radioactivity in relation to the wavelengths of illnesses that they have not attached any particular importance to the very powerful radioactivity of the water in Lourdes . . . I am not scared to declare that there are and will always be healings in Lourdes.[2]

In André Simoneton's opinion there were three principal factors at play in the healing properties of the waters at Lourdes:

- The physical state of the patient. To promote healing, the wavelength of his or her illness should "be synthesized" with that of this water.
- The psychic state of the patient. Faith, sustained through the practice of various rituals (including processions, songs, testimonies of miracles, and so on) over the course of his or her pilgrimage to Lourdes places the patient in a favorable state of receptivity—even if the patient is not a Catholic. (Miracles at Lourdes have also been known to have occurred to non-Catholics.)
- A third wave of limitless power, born from a phenomenon of resonance between the two previous waves. This permits the miracle to manifest—to immediately engender a "significant and profound change of the ill cells without destroying them . . . truly even to produce effects that we cannot even imagine."

As an example Simoneton cited a similar phenomenon that occurs in electricity:

> We know that the ampere wave has always shifted by a certain cosine phi with regard to the volt wave. If a resonance is produced between these two waves, by which I mean a superimposition of two waves of the same frequency, an extremely potent explosive power is created that will cause serious damage (such as disruption of a transformer or circuit breaker). It is to avoid these kinds of results that the cosine should always be as close as possible to its maximum interval—that is to say, the unit.[3]

We can imagine that a phenomenon of this order might be the cause—and thus the explanation for—the spectacular changes that have been observed occurring for certain patients at Lourdes.

As a final note, in 1973–1974, demonstrations revealed the existence of "neutral currents" involving neutrinos—particles that seem to exist as a transition between a material substance and biological phenomena. This was the basis for research by C. Louis Kervran on "transmutations by weak energy." It is this kind of transmutation that is at work in vitalized water (meaning water that is rich in metallic ions or minerals) as well as in the soil and among those plants capable of manufacturing elements that have not been supplied to them.

NATURAL AND PURIFIED WATERS

In its liquid state, water constitutes 50 to 75 percent of the weight of plants and 70 percent of the weight of the human body. It is easy to see the importance of the role it plays inside all living organisms. Natural water is generally mixed with mineral and organic "impurities," and is almost always tainted by dissolved gases (including carbon dioxide, CO_2). Water from mountains generally contains mineral salts, while as a rule water from the plains is less mineralized. Unfortunately, it is also often polluted by organic substances (albuminoid substances) that decay there, and by microorganisms.

MINERAL AND THERMOMINERAL WATERS

In its natural state, water is specifically categorized according to its dissolved salt content, temperature, and the gases of which it is composed. Because of their makeup, which includes trace elements, mineral waters generally have a beneficial effect in the treatment of certain illnesses. The deterioration of the therapeutic properties in mineral waters, upon being bottled, is probably due to the flocculation (see chapter 8, page 53) of a portion of their constituent ingredients. This is why better therapeutic results are obtained directly at the source of such waters than through drinking bottled mineral waters.

A spring is defined as thermomineral when its temperature is 5 Celsius degrees higher than the average temperature of the spring's above-ground environment. The majority of mineral waters have a temporary radioactivity (from radioactive bodies with a short life span, such as radon) and/or permanent radioactivity (from dissolved radium salts) that comes from the natural radioactivity of plutonic rocks like granite and some sedimentary rocks. The waters of a spa in Belgium, for instance, owe their radioactivity to that of the black schist of Stavelot.

Among the different substances in mineral waters, dissolved salts are the greatest in quantity, but they exist in a dissociated form that makes their reconstitution difficult. The results of chemical analysis of such waters are most often stated in a form based on ions. Among the anions these waters contain, chloride—which sometimes combines with iodine (as in the waters from Vichy, Bourbon-l'Archambault, Saratoga Springs, and French Lick) and bromine—is the most common and comes primarily from the dissociation of natural chlorides (halite and sylvine). Sulfur, generally in the form of sulfates, is a quite common constituent of these waters and originates either in the dissociation of sulfurs (pyrites) or sulfates (gypsum). Carbonic anions are quite often present as well. Fluorine can be found in many springs (Vichy, Luchon), whereas arsenic is much rarer (La Bourboule, Harbin Hot Springs). Among cations, sodium, often in combination with potassium, is the most widespread, principally in the form of chloride and sometimes as carbonate, bicarbonate, or sulfate. Calcium, accompanied or not by magnesium, can be found in a carbonate or chloride state. In fact, it is quite plentiful in some waters: 1.37 grams to the liter in the spring of Saint Allyre. Iron is present in almost all mineral waters in the form of carbonate or sulfate, whereas aluminum, lithium, barium, and strontium are much rarer. Substances that cannot be broken down also combine with the ions in these waters: boric acid, silicic acids, and colloids such as silica, sulfur, and ferric hydroxide. All of these elements are present from the leaching of the terrain in which the water circulates, though chemical and biochemical reactions can alter their ionic composition and their initial proportions along the way.

DIFFERENT TYPES OF THERMAL WATERS

It is customary to classify thermal waters into different types based on their dominant mineral composition:

- Lightly Mineralized Waters, which contain less than 500 mg of trace elements per liter (Hot Springs in Arkansas, Evian and Thonon-les-Bains in France)
- Bicarbonate Soda Waters (Vichy, Desert Hot Springs in California), Calcic Waters (Ussat), or Magnesiac Waters (Châtel)
- Chlorinated Waters (Saratoga Springs, Truth or Consequences in New Mexico, Salins-les-Bains, Salies-du-Salat)
- Sulfated Waters (Calistoga, Contrexéville, Capvern)
- Sulfured Waters (Berkeley Springs in West Virginia, Cauterets, Challes)

Thermal waters can also be classified based on their temperature when they emerge from the earth:
- Cold waters, less than 20° Celsius (Divonne-les-ains, Thonon-les-Bains)
- Hypothermal Waters, between 20° and 35° Celsius (Les Fumades, St. Honoré)
- Thermal Waters, between 35° and 50° Celsius (Barèges, Châteauneuf-les-Bains)
- Hyperthermal Waters, more than 50° Celsius (Dax, Amélie-les-Bains)
- Steam emissions (Yellowstone Park in Wyoming)

Thermal waters can also be categorized according to those trace elements that are richly present in their make-up:
- Arsenic (Harbin Hot Springs in California, La Bourboule, St. Honoré-les-Bains)
- Boron (Néris-les-Bains)
- Bromium (Gréoux-les-Bains, Challes-les-eaux)
- Copper (St. Christau, Castera-Verduzan)
- Iron (Harrogate in northern England, Aulus, Montrond, St. Christau, Marienbad)
- Fluorine (Beaucens, Vichy)
- Lithium (Néris-les-Bains, Amnéville, Ostend, Tehuacan in Mexico)
- Manganese (Uriage)
- Selenium (La Roche Posay)
- Silica (Desert Hot Springs, La Preste, Bains-les-Bains)
- Zinc (Uriage)

Because of the physicochemical variations (such as rechilling, decompression, oxidation, and various biological phenomena) at the outlets of the different springs, the substances they contain can either precipitate in the form of solid deposits (incrustations, concretions), or in the form of mud. Tufa and travertine formations are veritable rocks formed most often from aragonite, and more rarely from calcite, limonite, and gypsum. Silica is sometimes found in the form of opal, chalcedony, or quartz. Different kinds of mud that accumulate at the spots where thermomineral waters emerge consist largely of a blend of sediments and microorganisms (as at Aix-les-Bains).

LOOKING MORE CLOSELY AT THE CLASSIFICATION OF MINERAL WATERS

The most common way of classifying mineral waters is by their chemical composition. Based on the principal anion each water contains, different groups of waters are identified and divided according to the most prevalent cation. For example, carbonated waters, which are low in sulfate anions, can be found in areas that have recently experienced volcanic activity. These types are then further divided into sodic waters (such as those found at Mont Dore) or calcic waters (such as those at Bou Hanifa, Algeria). Even further delineation is possible: Chlorated waters, most often sodic, are frequently associated with Triassic rift and oil-bearing zones. Sulfated waters can be either calcic (Contrexéville) or sodic (Luxeil). Sodic sulfated waters constitute the majority of springs in the Pyrenees, whereas calcic sulfated waters are found in the Alps.

As indicated in the list above, thermal waters can also be classified based on temperature . In some spas the temperature of specific mineral waters is determined by the geothermal gradient. We should bear in mind, however, that because water cools as it rises, it must have a rapid ascent in order to retain its heat. Volcanic activity is another important source of heat (as shown by geysers in Iceland) as is cooling magma (as in Larderello, Italy) and, to a lesser extent, exothermic physicochemical reactions (such as the oxidation of iron pyrites) and the decay of radioactive bodies. Recently, hyperthermal waters have experienced a surge of renewed interest for the possibilities they offer as a source of heat for us. For example, several thousand inhabitants of the town of

HYDROXYDASE: AN EXCEPTIONAL MINERAL WATER

This uncommon mineral water is available only in certain health and specialty stores. (There are currently some fourteen U.S. distributors.) In addition to its extraordinarily high mineral content, it offers the undeniable advantage of being bottled in an airless vacuum so it reaches the hands of consumers still perfectly "alive," without having undergone standard preservative procedures. It should be drunk immediately when opened, which is why it is sold in small, 22 cc bottles which are easily finished.

Discovered in 1908 near Issoire (the Puy-de-Dôme department), it remains largely unknown to the public, yet it offers exceptional qualities thanks to the concentrations of minerals and various trace elements it contains. Analysis of this chloride bicarbonate water also reveals the presence of trace elements such as silver, lead, tin, nickel, and copper, and mineral salts such as magnesium, iron, calcium, sodium, and potassium. It is effective against all kinds of ailments and its high oxidoreduction potential makes it particularly practical in dealing with obesity and cellulite. Because it allows the destruction and elimination of toxins, it is also recommended for use in cases of arthritis, various kinds of poisoning, rheumatism, and even alcoholism.

Meulon in the Seine and Marne regions now get part of their heat from the hot waters in the Dogger aquifer.

A thermal or *thalassotherapy* cure fundamentally owes its effectiveness to the intake of natural and absorbable colloidal minerals and trace elements in conjunction with following various hydrotherapy practices, such as massage, bathing and showering, irrigating, steam bath inhaling, gargling, and so forth.

So ends this part of our investigation into colloidal minerals and trace elements. In the next part, we'll look much more closely at the roles of minerals and trace elements in the body.

PART 3

Minerals:
Building Blocks for Health

IO

THE BODY: A COMPOUND OF MINERALS AND TRACE ELEMENTS

The presence of trace elements in the primal sea and their catalytic and antioxydent properties have made them indispensable for the development of life. Much research has shown that the body is in fact a composite of colloidal minerals and trace elements.

As we learned earlier, fruits that have been cultivated in a soil that has been saturated with chemical fertilizers and pesticides have little taste or flavor. But fruits that have been grown naturally in soils that have not been chemically adulterated are charged with colloidal minerals, the very basis of life and of a healthy human body.

When the balance of colloidal minerals in the body is distorted, changed, or broken, minerals and trace elements are no longer pulled into the cells in the proper fashion. Instead they are deposited in the bones, nerves, and muscles, causing a kind of "scaling" that hardens the joints as well as nerves and muscles. These deposits are the source of various arthritic disorders, are a frequent cause of pain in the back and cervical regions, and are responsible for stiffness in the limbs and joints.

A COMPLETE MINERAL COCKTAIL

Minerals are indispensable to life in all its forms. Limiting, say, calcium and magnesium intake to the amount in daily supplements is quite insufficient for the body's needs. This is also true of iron, which is generally given as a supplement for women and children suffering from anemia. It is too often forgotten that when taken in its most commonly available medicinal form (which is nonorganic), iron can contribute to compromise of the body's hepatic functions.

What our bodies—and all living organisms—truly need is a very large cocktail of all the constituent minerals of our planet. These 92 elements are grouped together in the Periodic Table of Elements, also known as Mendelev's Periodic Chart (see fig. 10.1, page 92).

Based on the most current research available in this field, to maintain good health our bodies require the regular daily intake of at least 103 different nutrients: 72 minerals, 16 vitamins, 12 amino acids, and 3 essential fatty acids. Unfortunately it has become almost impossible to take in all of these just from the foods we eat.

These minerals and trace elements play various essential roles, depending upon their categorization:

- Some are involved in exchanges on the membranous level, the transmission of nerve impulses, and the supply of building elements to the bones.
- Some play a role in balancing the other elements—essential to maintaining a healthy immune system.
- Some form complexes with biological molecules according to an outline determined by the nature of the mineral or trace element, thereby enabling energy to adapt to a particular activity.
- Some facilitate specific biological processes by exchanging energy through the exchange of electrons.

It is easy to see that every element we take in is necessary and that the body cannot make do without any one of them or substitute one for another when a deficiency occurs. Not only is the presence of these minerals indispensable, but they also must be present in the necessary concentrations.

These elements exist inside the body in three different forms:

- As electrolytes they participate in maintaining osmotic pressure
- As transport elements they are affixed to proteins that deposit them in the tissues where they will either be used, stored, or eliminated.

Group	1	2	3	4	5	6	7	8	9	10	11	12	13	14	15	16	17	18
Period																		
1	1 H																	2 He
2	3 Li	4 Be											5 B	6 C	7 N	8 O	9 F	10 Ne
3	11 Na	12 Mg											13 Al	14 Si	15 P	16 S	17 Cl	18 Ar
4	19 K	20 Ca	21 Sc	22 Ti	23 V	24 Cr	25 Mn	26 Fe	27 Co	28 Ni	29 Cu	30 Zn	31 Ga	32 Ge	33 As	34 Se	35 Br	36 Kr
5	37 Rb	38 Sr	39 Y	40 Zr	41 Nb	42 Mo	43 Tc	44 Ru	45 Rh	46 Pd	47 Ag	48 Cd	49 In	50 Sn	51 Sb	52 Te	53 I	54 Xe
6	55 Cs	56 Ba	71 Lu	72 Hf	73 Ta	74 W	75 Re	76 Os	77 Ir	78 Pt	79 Au	80 Hg	81 Tl	82 Pb	83 Bi	84 Po	85 At	86 Rn
7	87 Fr	88 Ra	103 Lr	104 Rf	105 Db	106 Sg	107 Bh	108 Hs	109 Mt	110 Ds	111 Rg	112 Uub	113 Uut	114 Uuq	115 Uup	116 Uuh	117 Uus	118 Uuo

*Lanthanoids	57 La	58 Ce	59 Pr	60 Nd	61 Pm	62 Sm	63 Eu	64 Gd	65 Tb	66 Dy	67 Ho	68 Er	69 Tm	70 Yb
**Actinoids	89 Ac	90 Th	91 Pa	92 U	93 Np	94 Pu	95 Am	96 Cm	97 Bk	98 Cf	99 Es	100 Fm	101 Md	102 No

Fig. 10.1. The Periodic Table of Elements

Currently the table officially contains 109 chemical elements. The vertical columns group elements that have the same number of peripheral electrons in their atoms—meaning they have a similar chemistry—whereas the horizontal rows reflects an increasing number of protons (or electrons) present in the elements. It should be noted that in only one case are all the known isotopes of the same element grouped together, each of them differing from the others only in the number of neutrons at its core.

- As integral parts of proteins they can act as enzymatic cofactors or give proteins and nucleic acids their form. For example, we know of 200 enzymes that contain zinc, 4 that contain molybdenum, and more than 400 that contain magnesium.
- As components of hormones (such as thyroidal hormones)

SYNTHESIS OF DNA

Minerals play an essential role in the synthesis of DNA, the process of replication and duplication of cellular structures. In fact, the constant replacement of worn-out cells with new ones is entirely dependent upon trace elements. It is the body that determines what function a new cell will assume. The DNA molecule then programs it by providing it with genetic information in a way that ensures its proper functioning.

When a cell has not been programmed well because of a deficiency of essential nutrients, it will simply continue to exist without fulfilling its proper role; the cell is alive but simply does not know what to do. The ramifications of this are not great when only a few isolated, improperly functioning cells are scattered here and there, but when they accumulate in a specific location they may eventually form a tumor that could become cancerous. Or, when our bodies are no longer capable of consistently producing healthy cells, we may age prematurely or develop a number of diseases that could cause us to die before our time.

OUR ACID-ALKALINE BALANCE

It is also the responsibility of minerals to regularize our metabolism and maintain a balanced blood pH through their alkalinizing qualities,[1] which serve to buffer acids. As a general rule, our blood pH should remain slightly alkaline—between 7.35 and 7.45 on the pH scale. (We should recall that on the pH scale, acidity is indicated by readings lower than 7 and alkalinity by those higher than 7.) Outside of this ideal zone, at a highly acidic internal cellular environment of 6.8 or in extreme alkalosis at 8, our bodies no longer function optimally and our health deteriorates. If these limits are breached, the body experiences a metabolic breakdown that could lead to death.

THE DAMAGE CAUSED BY ACIDOSIS

Much research has shown that acidosis (a condition of reduced alkalinity of the blood and bodily tissues) is the source of aging, cardiovascular problems, cancer, and a large number of degenerative diseases. Of course, our bodies strive ceaselessly to maintain a correct acid-alkaline balance (pH). While a deficiency of essential minerals will push bodily fluids toward acidification, our cells—*anabolites*—secrete metabolic acid wastes called *catabolites*.

Anabolism is the activity that creates the building blocks of the body; in short, it is the transformation of nutritive substances into living tissue. Catabolism is the process consisting of the breakdown of the nutrients that are necessary for the creation of energy and the maintenance of life; it is essentially the transformation into energy of materials assimilated by the tissues. Catabolism, however, frees acids and can release them in excessive amounts, especially when we eat too many acidifying foods.

When the body is in an acidified state, the hematia—the red blood cells—use only 5 to 10 percent of their carrying capacity to transport oxygen to cells. The acids constantly generated by our metabolic functions must be quickly neutralized by alkaline minerals; if they are not, our teeth and bones may pay the consequences, and our natural immune system may well collapse. When this neutralizing cannot occur, or occurs insufficiently because of a mineral deficiency, decalcifications, osteoporosis, skin and hair problems, tooth decay, sciatica, depression, spasmophilia, muscle cramps, chronic fatigue, various digestive disorders, ulcerations, intestinal microlesions, anal burning, gingivitis, various allergies, conjunctivitis, recurring headaches, painful menstrual periods, cellular aging and so on are among the disorders that are likely to make an appearance.

THE THYMUS AND MINERALS

It is of vital importance that bodily fluids retain a slightly alkaline pH in order to protect the immune system. The thymus plays a major role in immunizing the body. It is this organ that produces the T cells (or *T lymphocytes*) that are responsible for protecting us against illness. During childhood the thymus occupies almost half of the thoracic cage. It begins to decrease in volume at around the age of twenty. At the age of sixty, it may be no more than 5 percent of its original size. When the percentage of T lymphocytes produced by the thymus begins to drop, a corresponding drop in immunity occurs. The body then begins to show a susceptibility to pathogens and viruses that produce opportunistic illnesses, which can become life threatening if the the body weakens sufficiently. As an example, the HIV detected in the blood transforms into AIDS only when the number of T lymphocytes falls.

Our bodies, at least as long as they are healthy and only to a certain point, are capable of effecting biotransformations—that is to say, transformations of toxins by enzymes so as to render them harmless. In order to be synthesized, these enzymes require the presence of numerous micronutrients, trace elements in particular. When these are missing, the machine breaks down because of insufficient cellular oxygenation. Toxins gain the upper hand . . . with all the health consequences that are observable today in the people who live in the West.

According to a survey taken in the 1980s by the head of the World Health Organization's department of research against cancer, Mr. John

MINIMIZING THE EFFECTS OF ACIDOSIS

Given the fact that the thymus increases in size within an alkaline environment and shrinks in size in an acidic environment, it is easy to see why it is an excellent idea to eat as many alkalizing foods as we can, but this alone will not always suffice to protect us from the effects of acidosis. Minerals play a key role in acid-alkaline balance—and are substances that are singularly lacking in our regular diet.

> [T]he fact that a number of illnesses can be cured simply by taking minerals is enough to show that mineral deficiency is a reality that must be taken into account in a world aware of the importance of nutrition despite the astounding progress of all kinds of disease that no one has been able to halt. The sole diet that is truly good for health is one that includes dietary supplements.*

———————————
*Dr. Robert R. Barefoot and Carl J. Reich, authors of the book *The Calcium Factor.*

Higgensen, "the elimination of 600 carcinogenic toxins present in the surrounding environment, in our air, water, and food, would be enough to prevent the manifestation of 90 percent of all cancers."

Knowing how unhealthy our world actually is, is it any surprise that our health is deteriorating and that as time passes this deterioration begins at a younger and younger age?

CELLULAR RESPIRATION

The cells that make up living organisms must be constantly renewed, yet the conditions of life today truly inhibit this kind of renewal. Every cell consists of various parts. In addition to the nucleus, which plays the role of the command center, it contains structures that make up an electrical center: ribosomes—which are responsible for, among other things, fabricating enzymes and albumin—and mitochondria, those nutritional structures that serve as generators of "fuel" for the cell through chemical reactions that free energy and effect the synthesis of certain proteins. Toxins in our system first attack the healthy functioning of the mitochondrion enzymes, essentially rendering the mitochondria inactive.

It is easy to see the domino effect established when, due ultimately to a lack of trace elements, the mitochondria's enzymes have been deactivated or their synthesis has been prevented. In the liver there are about 4000 mitochondria at work in a single cell! Through the process called cellular respiration, mitochondria transform glucose into energy in the presence of oxygen (hence the use of the term *respiration*). In addition to producing energy, they produce ATP (Adenosine triphosphate), a substance that comes into play in cellular metabolism, muscular contraction, and the synthesis of cortico-suprarenal gland hormones.

The process of cellular respiration is the source of the energy necessary for the life of the cell—and thus for the production of albumins or some 600 enzymes which, in turn, manufacture complex hormones and the antibodies that allow the body to defend itself against illnesses. For cellular respiration to take place in an optimal manner, numerous steps must play out. For example, oxygen can be used only when biocatalyzers (such as vitamins, minerals, and enzymes) are present. If these substances are lacking, the process breaks down. One result may be that we begin to feel tired and cold, or that we begin to experience other symptoms associated with old age. Aging is in part the result of a decline in cellular oxygenation, which is in turn connected to a tangible reduction of enzymes and a deficiency in vitamins and minerals.

It is essential, then, that we make the effort to maintain effective cellular respiration by taking in sufficient enzymes, amino acids, vitamins, and minerals. Because everything on our planet is interconnected, we are not alone in our dependence on cellular respiration. Also dependant on this process are the animals that supply us with food, the fish in our rivers and oceans, and the world's plants and trees. Damage to cellular respiration spells the eventual death of our forests, fish, and animals and the emergence of what we call "incurable" animal and human illnesses.

II
OUR HYDRO-MINERAL BALANCE

As we learned earlier, the colloidal state is a fundamental condition for living matter. It so happens that we are composed largely of water (about 72 percent), and it is within this nutritive water—in the form of colloidal solutions—that we find the minerals and trace elements that provide the material for our cells' fuel. The maintenance of a sound hydro-mineral balance, essential to our health if not our outright survival, is ensured by various body functions.

THE INTERNAL ENVIRONMENT

Every cell is constantly bathed in a complex colloidal solution that is our internal environment. The large quantity of water in this environment can be more or less significant with regard to tissue and organ function.

Living beings can be born, grow, and proliferate only to the extent that they meet a favorable ambient environment that includes, among other things, water and electrolytes, particularly potassium ($K+$), sodium ($Na+$), calcium ($Ca++$), and magnesium ($Mg++$) as cations, and chloride ($Cl-$) and phosphoric and sulfuric radicals as anions. From a strictly mineral point of view, what is known as the internal environment is the aqueous solution, of which 9 percent is made up of electrolytes. These mineral electrolytes are classified in two categories based on their concentration:

- Mineral salts whose concentration is higher than 1 ml per liter
- Trace elements whose concentration is lower than 1 ml per liter

In addition to minerals, the internal environment also consists of a group of organic fluids: lymph, blood plasma, and interstitial fluid, which together represent about 25 to 30 percent of the body's mass.

The internal environment supplies the body's cells with the substances it needs to live and function properly, and also permits it to get rid of its waste products. It is in fact the point of convergence for different regulatory systems of the body that interact to ensure the homeostasis of the internal environment, a dynamic balance that continually should be readjusting itself in response to changes tied to our environment and metabolism. It is this process of constant regulation on which the maintenance of osmotic pressure, pH, body temperature, blood sugar, and so forth depend. It is easy to see how important it is to maintain this balance. It is essential to health and even to life itself.

THE HYPOTHESIS OF THE STABILITY OF THE INTERNAL ENVIRONMENT, OR HOMEOSTASIS

The theory of the stability of the internal environment—proposed by Claude Bernard and restated by W. B. Cannon—can be summarized as follows: Among animals an entire series of processes comes into play to maintain the stability of the internal environment's chemical composition and its physiochemical characteristics when there are changes in the environment.

The absolute nature of this hypothesis, however, has not shielded it from some major criticisms. This extremely fertile, seductive, and stimulating theory was formulated at a time when variability was viewed as an error and its foreseeable temporal nature was completely ignored. A new concept of the regulation of the internal environment also takes into account biological rhythms.

EXCHANGES

When studying the hydro-electrical (or hydro-mineral) metabolism, the physiologist analyzes the exchanges that can be seen at every level of the organization of living beings. These exchanges exist in all living things—within single-celled organisms, plants, and the most evolved forms of animal life. Among these latter, exchanges can be found at every stage of the anatomic structure from the subcellular and cellular level to the level of the body as a whole.

The notion of hydro-electrical exchanges between each cell and extracellular fluids cannot be disassociated from the notion of exchanges of water and mineral substances that take place between an entire organism and the ambient environment. R. Quinton (1897) and A. B. MacCallum (1903) advanced the idea that seawater may well have been the original ambient environment of living things. Interestingly, it is true that the extracellular fluids of highly organized animals have a composition reminiscent of seawater (high in sodium and chloride, low in potassium).

Exchanges between an organism and its environment or between the different parts of an organism may be explained in terms of mineral metabolism. This is an important subject, for it has been observed that if the redistribution of a cellular or extracellular component occurs for a significant and prolonged period of time, disorders of varying seriousness and intensity are likely to follow. Many of the symptoms of specific physical ailments are in fact linked to disturbance of the natural redistribution of water and electrolytes.

REDISTRIBUTION OF WATER AND ELECTROLYTES

It is essential that water and electrolytes be unevenly distributed in the body. Any alteration of this arrangement, beyond certain limits, will lead to death.

Water and ions play irreplaceable roles in a long series of biochemical and biophysical mechanisms, including maintenance of cellular hydration (balanced osmotic pressure between intracellular liquids—ICL—and extracellular liquids—ECL), participation in numerous enzymatic processes, and intervention in the metabolizing of glucids and protids. Some displacement of $K+$, $Na+$, $Ca++$, and $Mg++$ ions are also closely linked to cerebral, nervous, muscular, cardiac, and glandular activities.

To get a good picture of the uneven nature of water and electrolyte distribution throughout an organism, we can imagine the body as being made up of several spaces, sectors, or compartments that are separated from one another by membranes, with the environment of each space consisting of a number of well-defined fluids: extracellular liquids that are quite high in $Na+$ and $Cl-$ and intracellular liquids that are very high in $K+$ and phosphoric radicals. While this general mix is found in both plant and animal organisms, there are differences among species as well as among organ types inside the internal cellular environment of the same species. In fact, knowing that osmotic pressure here is proportionate to the molecular concentration of the ions present, any change in the concentration of a single constituent of one of these environments is accompanied by a change in its osmotic pressure. The outcome can be a transfer of water through the walls provoking a swelling or a retraction of cells. Accordingly, when an exogenous intake of sodium chloride increases the concentration of ECL, a transfer of water from the cells to the space around it tends to correct this gap.

VARIATIONS IN BIOLOGICAL CONSTANTS

The majority of values in the tables of biological constants can give only a general idea of the actual distribution of ions. This estimate must be supplemented by an estimate of the relative variability of intra- and extracellular liquids.

The amount of the dose used does not provide any information on the biological properties of the mineral under consideration. For example, while 43 percent of the total sodium in the body is concentrated in the bones, only three tenths of this bone $Na+$ is actually exchangeable. The remaining seven tenths is non-exchangeable, belonging to the bone structure itself.

We also know that water in the body exists in at least two forms: the free or circulating water that behaves like a solvent and that can be found in blood and lymph, and bound water, in particular the colloidal water we take in, which, when fixed to proteins, acquires a distinctive resistance to evaporation and the process of congealing. The actual calculation of exchangeable $Na+$, $K+$, or $Ca++$ is relatively difficult to determine.

It has also been observed that hydration diminishes with age in human beings and other mammals. Expressed as a percentage of total body mass, water represents 93 percent of the weight of a four-month-old fetus, 85 percent of that of a seven-month-old premature baby, 80 percent of that of a newborn, and 72 percent of a young and healthy adult. This percentage continues to fall throughout our lifetime—sometimes reaching as low as 60 percent in the very elderly, who, as a result, run the risk of dehydration, especially in the event of summer heat waves.

The amount of each mineral in units of weight in the body also varies considerably from birth to maturity. Between these two ages, the amount of Na+ decreases by 1.7 times, and Cl- by 1.3. Meanwhile, K+ and Ca++, two intracellular elements, will increase proportionately 1.5 and 2.2 times their current measurements, respectively.

Modern research has revealed that the hydro-electrolytic constitution of extra- and intracellular fluids is far from stable. Instead, it varies in a rhythmic and predictable way. There is evidence of circadian metabolic rhythms (with periods of roughly 24 hours), at every level of organization in living beings. The circadian variations of hydro-electrolytic metabolism represent a significant part of the temporal structure of organisms.

THE ROLE OF CELLULAR MEMBRANES

The most abundant cations in the body are calcium (Ca), magnesium (Ma), sodium (Na), potassium (K), and phosphorus (P). While sodium is characteristic of the extracellular internal environment, potassium is specifically found in intracellular fluid. The composition of the salts found in intra- and extracellular fluids are different although they are dependent upon each other. Exchanges are ensured by the ion pumps of the cellular membrane.

Cellular membranes are more or less an obstacle for the entry or exit of one or more ions. Passage through a living membrane is defined as a *passive transport* when it is the direct consequence of the effects of physical forces working on specific ions; these physical forces can result from:

- A movement of water, which leads to the dissolution of substances
- A difference in concentration
- A difference in the electrical potential between the two sides of the membrane

An ion will move from an area where the force is most intense toward where it is weakest. This is what is known as passive transport. *Active transport* (or ascending transport), on the other hand, occurs when there is no physical force acting on the ions. This type of ion movement is possible only in the presence of energy that has been taken in and stored in the cell.

COMPENSATION FOR LOSSES FROM INTAKE OF WATER AND MINERAL SALTS

All living things must compensate for biological losses. Everyday we experience loss of water and mineral salts. On average, the per-day requirements for every adult human in good health are:

- about 2.7 liters of water
- 50 to 125 mEq (milliequivalent) of potassium
- 50 to 150 mEq of sodium
- 50 to 150 mEq of chloride

Absorption of these occurs primarily through the digestive tract, principally through the small intestine. This absorption is rapid, efficient, and intense. Elimination chiefly occurs through the kidneys as urine and, secondarily, through other wastes such as feces and sweat.

It is noteworthy that in fish the amount of Na+ excreted is more significant from the gills than from the kidneys. Similarly, tortoises, penguins, and seagulls possess nasal glands capable of ensuring a very effective nonrenal elimination of sodium chloride. It is so effective, in fact, that these creatures can absorb seawater without suffering any ill effects.

Our different hormones play a role in the regulation of these elements. For example, the hormones of the cortico-suprarenal gland—aldosterone, cortisol, and cortisone—encourage the body to retain sodium and eliminate potassium. Their action takes place largely in the kidneys, but they also act on digestive absorption and on the cellular distribution of potassium, calcium, and sodium.

Other hormones such as adrenaline, noradrenaline, growth hormone, prolactins, thyroid hormones, androgens, progesterone, and insulin can also influence hydro-electric metabolism within the bounds of a circadian rhythm.

THE INTERACTION AND
EQUILIBRIUM OF MINERALS

As we have seen through the course of this book, our bodies require not one mineral salt in particular but a cocktail made from all minerals. There is no mineral that works independently of the others; all interact directly or indirectly with each of the other electrolytes. For example, magnesium can be absorbed effectively only when a balanced calcium-phosphorus liaison is present. And a proper balance of magnesium and sodium depends upon a normal rate of potassium intake. This interdependence can be observed with all the electrolytes.

This does not suggest that it is a good idea for people to take excessive quantities of non-organic mineral supplements. Studies have shown that though the body will utilize a supplement in the case of a specific mineral need (such as a crisis of spasmophilia), 10 to 20 times more than the organic form of the mineral is required in order to achieve the same results. Such high dosages, however, are not easy for the body to assimilate and present the risk of an overdose that in and of itself can have adverse consequences.

How, then, should we address our need for supplements? First, we should take supplements in a form that is measurable and easily assimilated by the body—in other words, in a form that the body recognizes as food, such as chelated substances presented in a vegetable protein base. Remember, we are unable to assimilate minerals directly and, in order to meet our needs, must use intermediaries in the plant kingdom.

As for the trace elements we require, materials that not only are essential to the body's smooth functioning, but also ensure the better utilization of those minerals we take in larger doses through diet or through balanced supplements: It is rare to find a "prescription" that contains the entire range of known trace elements. Many of them are not even available in pharmacies, and legislation concerning their availability varies from one country to the next. Ideally we should take trace elements in the form of a complex in synergy with plant extracts (there are a number of these currently offered on the market), in the naturally occurring form of a colloidal water of plant origin (such as the spring that serves as the source for T. J. Clark's products), or, as is the case with Quinton's Marine Plasma, as a solution whose source is the ocean.

12
COLLOIDAL MINERALS: SPARKS OF LIFE

The body "homeopathicizes" the medication and it is only
to the extent that such a "homeopathicification" occurs
that any therapeutic action is achieved.
VICTOR BOTT, *SPIRITUAL SCIENCE AND*
THE ART OF HEALING: RUDOLF STEINER'S
ANTHROPOSOPHICAL MEDICINE

OUR BODIES ARE
ELECTRICAL CENTERS

Certainly it is possible to describe water as an energy harnesser and high-frequency oscillator, but our bodies, too, are a kind of electrical center. Everyone knows what happens when the power to our homes or offices is cut: All of a sudden we find ourselves in the dark and nothing will run. In fact, without electricity, our modern world shuts down completely. In simple terms, all we need to do is flick a switch to create electricity at the voltage necessary to feed all our electrical appliances. The situation is much the same in the body.

COLLOIDAL MINERALS
FROM NATURAL SOURCES

Organic colloidal minerals are the essential sparks of life that generate and maintain electrical production in our bodies. The body is dependent on these minerals for literally tens of thousands of biochemical functions. In order for our bodies to stay switched on and healthy, these vital nutrients must be constantly replenished. For instance, a lack of electrolyte elements (sodium, potassium, and chloride) can cause fatigue, muscle weakness, and electrical disturbances to the heart. Electrical disturbances to the heart can result in erratic, rapid, or skipped heartbeats, or [the heart may] simply stop beating all together.[1]

As we have seen, microorganisms present in the soil transform inorganic minerals into a form that can be utilized by plants. Plants absorb these minerals through their roots and by virtue of photosynthesis transform them into carbon-based organic molecules. A mineral molecule of plant origin is a microscopic particle about 0.0001 micron in diameter, about one six hundredth the size of a red blood cell. Their size in colloidal mineral complexes of plant origin is the main reason why the body can easily utilize them to maintain the bioelectrical balance that is essential to health and longevity and to improve the availability and assimilation of other nutrients, such as vitamins from food and other dietary supplements.

Studies of that rich spring water from Utah,* undertaken in the Ana-Bio Corp Laboratories with the help of an argon plasma spectroscope, have revealed the presence of an extremely wide spectrum of seventy-two minerals, including rare trace elements and an additional twenty hyper trace elements in an electro-colloidal form. And similarly, in seawater we can find all ninety-two elements in the Periodic Table—all in a form that is easily assimilated by the cells in proportions that are fairly close to those encountered in the internal cellular environment of the body.

The role of electrocolloidal elements in biochemical and bioelectrical reactions has only recently been established, first for plants, then for humans and animals. Colloidal trace elements are the essential catalysts

---

*Available commercially from the T. J. Clark company.

for a number of metabolic functions. By their presence alone they trigger or re-ignite chemical reactions that will not take place in their absence, mainly because the initial signal is electrical in nature, in the blue-violet band of the spectrum, demonstrated German physicist Fritz-Albert Popp, who first conceived of Light Biology. Polarized with a negative electrical charge, colloidal substances attract toxins and poisons, which they aid in removing from our cells at the same time that they deposit the mineral or mineralloid substances they bring into the cells. In this way, they reactivate cellular function and help to strengthen the immune system.

The most advanced studies in biophysics and in molecular biochemistry have shown that minerals play a critical role in the synthesis of DNA and RNA, which are the foundations of the replication and duplication of the cellular structure. Deficiencies and subdeficiencies in electrocolloidal trace elements will cause the processes of cellular regeneration to dysfunction and abort. As a result, we age more quickly, develop all kinds of chronic diseases—which in turn are maintained by iatrogenic action of chemical medicines—and we die before our time.

ENZYMES AND COLLOIDAL MINERALS

As we have seen, enzymes, those indispensable proteins, are the catalysts that encourage and accelerate chemical-biological reactions. More than 3,000 enzymes that are indispensable for metabolic function have been identified. The importance of the role played by these enzymes and catalysts in fundamental physiological mechanisms is well known. Yet despite the fact that all the body's metabolic functions, including the digestion and assimilation of the food we eat and the initiation of all cellular functions, is dependent upon enzymes, most people lack these necessary substances.

Enzymes can be synthesized only when certain micronutrients, including metals, trace amounts of metalloids, and colloidal minerals, are present. In mineral chemistry, metals are catalysts. Enzymes, for their part, most often possess one metal atom in their active grouping—a metal that plays a role in the mechanical process of the reaction. Colloidal minerals, like trace elements, enter into the composition of all enzymes or are involved in the numerous reactions these enzymes initiate. We know, for example, that colloidal magnesium is an essential element involved in the composition of numerous enzymes that govern a large number of physiological functions. The Krebs Cycle, in which specific enzymes play a role at every stage, is one of the better known examples.*

SYNTHESIS OF HORMONES

Minerals and trace elements also play a major role in the synthesis of different hormones and in the regulation of the entire endocrine system, which consists of the thyroid, the parathyroids, the pineal gland, the pancreas, the ovaries, the testicles, the thymus gland, the suprarenal gland, and the pituitary gland. It is easy to imagine the fairly significant, varied, and numerous repercussions of any potential deficiencies in this system. These would include hormonal disorders of all kinds, sterility, fatigue, lowered immune system, insomnia, diabetes, and osteoporosis.

VITAMINS

We know that vitamins are complex chemical substances indispensable to nutrition, and that each of them is of importance for the normal function of a specific structure in the body. We know that disorders and disease result from any vitamin deficiency. But it is not commonly realized that vitamins control the body's appropriation of minerals, and that therefore in the absence of minerals they have no function to perform. Lacking vitamins, the system can make some use of minerals, but lacking minerals, vitamins are useless.[2]

Minerals are also essential for metabolizing the vitamins that are crucial for health and for ensuring their optimum utilization by the body. Few of us may be aware, for instance, that the body cannot assimilate vitamin E without the proper amount of colloidal zinc in the bloodstream. Likewise, as many of us now know, the presence of Vitamin D is essential for the assimilation of calcium, and Vitamin C is necessary for the absorption of iron.

---

*The Krebs Cycle is a series of intracellular enzymatic reactions that produce energy during the time it takes for glucids to decay.

COLLOIDAL MINERALS ARE NEVER TOXIC

It is important to stress that, unlike minerals and metals of nonorganic origin, colloidal minerals are never toxic. For example, drinking the equivalent of two teaspoons of iodine is likely to be fatal—which makes Dr. Frederic Macy's story that much more significant. Macy was a highly regarded bacteriologist who had an extensive understanding of colloidal chemistry. He explained the workings of colloids in the body in this way:

> The effect of colloids is explainable in part by electric action. Sick and dead and broken-down cells are attracted to the colloids by electromagnetic force, as iron filings are attracted to a magnet. The colloids carry those decayed or poisonous substances into the blood stream, and they are eliminated, the system meanwhile adapting what it needs of the colloids.[3]
>
> During a demonstration, Dr. Macy drank an entire glass of iodine, an amount capable of killing three hundred people. He then explained that the metals and minerals normally considered toxic were in fact poisonous only when they existed in a "free" state. In colloidal form, however, not only were they nontoxic, they were actually beneficial. During this demonstration he showed that iodine in a colloidal state offered absolutely no danger whatsoever.[4] (Despite the fact that Dr. Macy's demonstration showed the harmlessness of iodine in a colloidal state, readers are nevertheless advised not to attempt to duplicate his experiment, which could be fatal if not carried out correctly.)

HEAVY METALS

Like iodine, arsenic, lead, aluminum, and mercury—all of which are highly toxic and/or fatal in their normal state—can be beneficial in a colloidal state.

Colloidal aluminum is present in all plants, including those that are edible. It is one of the most abundant minerals found in soil. Many scientists believe colloidal aluminum from plants is an essential element of human nutrition. Of course, aluminum remains the subject of much controversy today, in particular for being implicated as a possible player in Alzheimer's disease. Regarding this concern, a communiqué from Harvard University, however, states that the scientific research on this subject never specifies which form of aluminum has been questioned—seemingly a significant point. And a study conducted at Oxford University has shown that the same percentage of aluminum is found in the brains of both Alzheimer's patients and those who do not suffer from the disease.

Colloidal arsenic is essential for the survival of newborns. Based on tests of rats from whose diet arsenic was eliminated, a study has established that their growth rate slowed considerably, they lost their fur, and they seldom moved. Their red blood cells had become almost completely inactive. When arsenic in a colloidal state was introduced, the opposite effects were produced and their energy level improved spectacularly.

Colloidal minerals from natural sources do not collect in the body and thus do not produce levels of toxicity. In fact, they attract heavy metals such as mercury, lead, and other toxic substances present in the body and encourage their elimination.

13
THE ROLE OF
TRACE ELEMENTS

It seems clear that, with respect to living matter, the elements of construction and combustion that are present in larger quantities (such as sodium, calcium, potassium, phosphorus, carbon, oxygen, and nitrogen) can be organized only when accompanied by elements that are much rarer and infinitesimal in quantity, and are present only to permit the reactions necessary for life: the trace elements.

GABRIEL BERTRAND,
LES ELEMENTS BIO-CATALYTIQUES

TRACE ELEMENTS AND
RARE EARTHS

Let us start this chapter by recalling that these mineral substances (metals and metalloids) are present in very small quantities in all living organisms. They represent only .001 percent of body mass, which translates into about .25 ounce for a person weighing 150 pounds! They play an essential biological role, however, and are indispensable to plant, animal, and human life.

Trace elements can generally be divided into two groups:

- Essential or major trace elements, which include iron, calcium, magnesium, zinc, copper, and silicon.
- Minor trace elements, including hyper-trace elements such as selenium, vanadium, manganese, cobalt, nickel, chromium, and iodine.

Rare earths are those minor trace elements that are necessary in even smaller proportions. Among these are lanthanum, praseodymium, neodymium, samarium, europium, ytterbium, yttrium, and thulium. Although it is not yet possible to determine the precise effects of each trace element, studies seem to show that they do in fact double an animal's life expectancy in the laboratory.

The human body contains all the elements of the Periodic Table that are available to it in its environment. Some of these elements are termed essential because their absence is incompatible with life and their deficiency engenders specific pathological conditions. Nevertheless, it remains true that all elements are necessary for our equilibrium, even those that occur only as traces or hyper-traces.

Though extreme deficiencies are rare in our modern Western world, lesser deficiencies are plentiful enough to fill our hospital wards. Yet it has been observed repeatedly that simply taking a supplement of elements that we are missing is often enough to correct the presenting problem. The body is perfectly capable of choosing what it needs, regulating even infinitesimal quantities provided it has been given the greatest possible selection of trace elements—which amounts to a daily dose of biocolloidal complexes such as those discussed in chapter 12.

Just like minerals, trace elements play precise roles in all our biological processes:

- They act as enzymatic cofactors because of their electronic structure, which permits them to possess several levels of oxidation.
- They act as hormonal cofactors.
- They play a role in the composition of vitamins (such as vitamin B12).
- They are necessary to the composition of structural proteins (membranous tubulines).
- They stabilize the structure of the nucleotides in nucleic acids.
- They enter into the composition of all our tissues—organs,

muscle, bone, bodily fluids, and so forth—and take part in all the exchanges that permit sound cellular functioning.

- They are catalysts at play in many bodily functions and reactions that could not either take place or be completed without their presence.
- Their action is very specific, precise, and related to a determined chemical activity.
- They boost the immune system, fight free radicals, and improve the internal cellular environment, thereby encouraging the body's natural defenses.
- They encourage all metabolic exchanges, such as respiration and nutrition.
- They are essential for hormonal regulation as well as for the renewal of body tissue. Zinc, for instance, helps to regulate testosterone and acts in the synthesis of prostaglandins while selenium plays a role in the regulation of thyroid hormones.

In short, trace elements are the major agents in the biochemistry of living things, whether plants, animals, or humans.

THE IMPORTANCE OF VERY SMALL QUANTITIES

The physiological effects of trace elements can vary considerably depending on the amount taken in. Calcium serves as a good example: When taken in an ionized form, calcium has coagulant properties. Taken in large doses it will therefore restore calcium to depleted bone or tissue. In very small amounts provided in colloidal form, however, it is endowed with regulating properties.

ELEMENTS IN THE HUMAN BODY

We now know that all of the elements in the following list play a role in the composition of the human body. It should be noted that the list is not exhaustive and that the importance of additional elements will likely be determined in the future.

aluminum	antimony	arsenic	barium
beryllium	boron	bromine	cadmium

calcium	carbon	cerium	cesium
chloride	chromium	cobalt	copper
fluoride	germanium	gold	hydrogen
indium	iodine	iron	lead
lithium	magnesium	manganese	mercury
molybdenum	nickel	nitrogen	oxygen
phosphorus	potassium	rubidium	samarium
scandium	selenium	silicon	silver
sodium	strontium	sulfur	tantalum
thallium	thorium	tin	titanium
tungsten	uranium	vanadium	zinc

When nature combines these elements in exact proportions, the result is a living, breathing, functioning human being who, once crafted out of these materials, will continue to regenerate for the rest of his or her life. In order for this to occur, however, it is essential that we constantly receive these same elements, which continue to be precisely combined so that each of us can realize his or her full potential emotionally and physically.

Chemist Justus Liebig made an important observation that was echoed by Schussler and subsequently confirmed in 1918 by Dr. Wessberge in his doctoral thesis presented to the Sorbonne: These elements can enter our cells only in small amounts that have been extremely diluted. "If fragments of nervous tissue are immersed in solutions of the same salt, but in increasing concentrations, the following two results can be observed:

1. The less salt in the solution, the more quickly it is assimilated and its effect accentuated.
2. When the quantity of salt in the solution exceeds a certain amount, the opposite phenomenon occurs: Instead of assimilating it, the immersed tissue retracts, loses weight, and rapidly putrefies."[1]

As Liebig noted, when the mineral substances necessary to a plant are provided in too large a quantity, the plant eventually dies. A mineral substance that encourages a plant's growth when present in small amounts may adversely affect or even kill it when presented in quantities that are too great. The same seems to be true for animals and humans.

By way of illustration, though a billionth of a gram of metal contains 2.5 billion atoms, it takes only 10 atoms on average to reactivate an enzyme molecule. Carboxypeptidase (human cytocuprein) contains 2 atoms g/mol. As an example, we can look at copper. The enzyme's activity is optimal between 200 and 240 g/mol of copper, diminishes at 240 to 400 g/mol, and simply drops off completely at 675 g/mol.

ANOTHER EXPERIMENT PERFORMED BY L. KOLISKO

Other experiments of this nature were performed by L. Kolisko[2] during Rudoph Steiner's lifetime and according to his instructions. Some wheat seeds were placed in a potentized homeopathic solution of metallic salts to germinate as test subjects, while others were placed in distilled water as control subjects. It was then observed that the lower potentizations—1X, 2X, 3X—had a paralyzing effect on the growth of the sprouts—an effect that was mitigated as the rate of potentization was increased until growth reached, eventually, a 0 value, at which point the sprouts exhibited no difference from the control subjects. When the experiment was continued with greater dilutions, an acceleration of the growth process was observed, which, after reaching a maximum, decreased until a 0 value was again reached, after which growth was increasingly restrained. These experiments have often been repeated, always with the same results.[3]

Since the time of Kolisko's experiments, a number of other researchers have shown interest in the effects of metallic salts on bodily processes. Among these we can cite the work of Jarricot, Bertrand, Person, Devraigne, Boiron, Wurmser, Lapp and still be far from exhausting the list. The findings of Kolisko's study opened the way to further research on trace elements and the properties of colloidal minerals.

OLIGOTHERAPY: A MEDICINE FOR THE BODY'S INTERNAL CELLULAR ENVIRONMENT

Toward the end of the nineteenth century and at the beginning of the twentieth, a time rich with discovery, Gabriel Bertrand propelled biochemistry forward by supplying evidence of the key role played by metal and metalloid biocatalysts, even those present in very small amounts. In fact, it was he who first coined the term *trace elements*. During his lifetime he studied the elementary composition of living tissues and the chemical transformations characteristic of their biological activity. His work also focused on diastases (now known as enzymes), mainly on the oxydases. He discovered the role of trace elements in enzymatic activity within living cells and, in 1894, proposed the hypothesis that metallic elements played the essential roles of coenzymes. (It should be noted that in current scientific terminology the word *coenzyme* is used to designate two very different types of enzymatic factors.)

Maurice Javillier made his own decisive discoveries on phosphorus, magnesium, and the catalytic elements. With Raulin and Pasteur, he contributed evidence of the considerable influence of trace minerals on the development of microorganisms, thereby leading the discovery that a complete deficiency of manganese prevented development in molds and that animals were also sensitive to this deficiency, which prompted degeneration of the testicular germinative tissue and other pathological disorders.

Once the physiological effects of biocatalysts had been grasped, it was possible to move on to their therapeutic applications. In 1932 Jacques Ménétrier, using Gabriel Bertrand's research as his base, began to envision the immense possibilities offered by the application of trace elements in human medicine. He refined solutions for those trace elements that were identified at the time and defined an original therapeutic method, which of course led to difficulties with those who upheld conventional medicine. Despite his condemnation by the Council of the Order of Doctors in 1954, his method utilizing biocatalysts went on to enjoy widespread success, even though he, its originator, remained in the shadows.

OLIGOTHERAPY AND CHAOS THEORY

According to chaos theory, when a system finds itself close to demarcation between two states, it takes only a trifling event to force the transition from one state to another. A similar theory called the butterfly effect has been articulated by the physicist Konrad Lorenz: By merely beating its wings a butterfly may be responsible for generating a hurricane on the other side of the globe. Chaos theory actually lends great support to Ménétrier's hypothesis by allowing for great flexibility in the substance of biochemical reactions as well as for their immediate adaptation to conditions imposed by the environment.

We may look at the example of a person suffering from an allergic internal cellular environment at the whim of environmental conditions. Because of this, the individual constantly shifts between health and allergic disorders. It seems possible in these circumstances that repeated microdoses of certain trace elements would permit the internal cellular environment to stabilize and thus prevent its habitual reactivity to allergic stimuli.

In his theory Ménétrier classified his patients based on a series of symptoms that were grouped according to the different internal cellular environments caused by functional deficiencies. As he saw it, these deficits had to be connected to disturbances of certain enzymatic sequences marked by a deficiency in certain trace elements or groups of trace elements. He surmised that small doses of these missing trace elements would thus serve as a signal to trigger corrective reactions. In order for this theory to test positively, it was necessary, of course, that there be no corresponding deficiency of one or more of the so-called essential trace elements. Also to be avoided in all subjects was oxidative stress, which has as its source the body's anarchic and uncontrolled production of free radicals.

Oxidative Stress

Oxidative stress is a result of the cell's physiological response to attack, which can take the form of too much sun or too much junk food or a prolonged exposure to adrenaline or the advance of a virus or bacteria. When under assault, the cell reacts through oxidation (the loss of electrons from electron-rich chemical bonds during a chemical reaction) and the production and release of oxidated free radicals. If this response is excessive, however, or if the body's regulating systems have broken down, the cell then finds itself attacked by its own production of free radicals, which results in damage to the cellular membrane.

One of the keys to regulating the production of free radicals is an enzyme called superoxyde dismutase in which three essential trace elements can be found: manganese, copper, and zinc. Other protective enzymes include glutathione peroxydase (which contains selenium) and catalase (which contains manganese). Free radicals do, of course, play an important role in the overall workings of the body (they help carry electrons and take part in the various mechanisms of synthesis inside the cell), but only when they exist in the appropriate proportions—proportions that are quickly exceeded by all kinds of factors in modern life. The job of the trace elements—particularly selenium—is to inhibit the production of free radicals while protecting the lipidic portion of the cellular membrane.

Many aspects of the complex mechanisms involving trace elements still remain unexplained, but research is ongoing—particularly in the area of the interactions between enzymes and trace elements.

Diathesis

Diathesis is the classification of basic constitutional pathological tendencies established by Ménétrier from studies he conducted with his patients. He believed that the internal cellular environment can be broken down into five types:

- Allergic Diathesis. The subject is hyper-reactive, subject to acute reactions and symptoms that appear and develop capriciously. This patient often suffers from tachycardia, precordial chest pains, seasonal asthma and hay fever, gastritis or food intolerance, rheumatic pains accompanied by inflammation, migraines, or hormonal problems (dysmenorrhea, dysthyroidia). The specific treatment for this type of internal cellular environment is manganese.
- Hypostenic Diathesis. The subject tires easily, is lacking in strength, and requires a great deal of sleep. He or she works slowly and needs a calm, unruffled setting. Physical problems manifest mainly in respiration, within the thoracic cavity and in the ORL (Otitis, Rhino, Laryngitis) sphere. People in this category may also suffer from tooth decay and cavities, eczema, infected acne, ligamentary hyperlaxity, infectious colitis, or constipation. Treatments are manganese and copper.
- Dystonic Diathesis. The subject exhibits a marked slowing down. Asthenia (abnormal loss of strength) becomes constant, accompanied by anxiety and, quite often, insomnia. The various

symptoms are all akin to a neurovegetative dystonia: irregular heartbeat, dizziness, tinnitus, nonallergic asthma, gastric spasms, spasmodic colopathies, and early stage osteoarthritis. Treatment consists of manganese and cobalt.

- Anergic Diathesis. Asthenia becomes intense and permanent in the subject and is often accompanied by disgust with life and psychic and physical aboulia (loss of will power). Depression is quite possible. Of course, the overwhelming sense of being defeated weakens the immune system's defenses, which leads to the risk of a number of disorders if no steps are taken to address the situation. Specific treatment consists of copper, gold, and silver.

- Maladaptation of the Endocrine System. This condition will accompany the other diatheses and add functional disorders related to the endocrine system, most particularly those of a hypophysary nature. A zinc-copper combination will regulate this kind of dysfunction, which is often accompanied by sexual asthenia and neurohormonal problems during adolescence or during menopause or andropause (decrease in male hormones). A zinc-nickel-cobalt combination is effective in the case of a hypophyso-pancreatic imbalance with digestive manifestation, characterized by irregular sensations of complete exhaustion, sudden cravings for food, and a temporary decrease of the intellectual faculties.

The categorizing of diatheses allows for the grouping of different and sometimes seemingly conflicting symptoms that all have the same fundamental cause. It also makes it possible to plot the therapeutic context. As Michel Deville explains:

> Diathesis expresses generally the transition between the healthy state and the lesional syndrome (or group of elementary lesions) . . . A secondary pathological attack is physiologically the consequence of a growing anomaly in the body's exchanges and a progressively larger blockage of its regulating functions.[4]

Of course there is no such thing as a pure diathesis; it is simply a convenient classification that aids in addressing a physical condition.

Each diathesis corresponds to a type of physical behavior and intellectual and psychological characteristic that tend to exhibit certain

WHAT IS A BIOCATALYST?

Catalysis is a chemical phenomenon in which certain bodies called catalysts, in very small amounts, accelerate chemical reactions and sometimes even encourage one reaction over another though the substance acting as a catalyst may not undergo any permanent change. Biocatalysis, connected to biochemistry, the chemistry of life, can be defined as the action of biocatalysts within living tissue, where they encourage the chemical reactions that are essential to life. Among the biocatalysts considered indispensable for maintaining life are vitamins, minerals, hormones, and enzymes.

In the biological sphere (according to the research of Berzélius in 1835), when a substance has available several different possible paths to take, the biocatalyst will accelerate the only reaction that protects the integrity of the tissue.

symptoms. Each diathesis also corresponds to one of the five elements of Traditional Chinese Medicine, and therefore to one or more organs as well as to the various characteristics attributed to each of these five elements.

Treatment using trace elements—or oligotherapy—essentially involves the body's internal cellular environment and addresses the roots of illness rather than its symptoms. Oligotherapy works on the level of cellular and tissular exchanges themselves in order to restore balance to these exchanges. In turn, the body's natural defenses will be strengthened. While trace elements can be used to address certain benign symptomological conditions (many people, for instance, have experienced the benefits of copper when fighting off the flu), they are extremely effective in treatment at a much deeper level.

OUR TRACE ELEMENT NEEDS

Determining the supplement that will meet out needs depends on what we are actually getting in our regular diet—not just what we are taking in, but also the bioavailability of these elements. Remember, our ability to assimilate them can be disrupted by a number of factors. We should be aware that in the event that we are experiencing a deficiency in a particular substance, the effects it causes will appear only gradually. In fact, it is possible that they may exist unnoticed, hidden behind various symptoms that may be all too readily attributed to a specific disease or condition with which they are normally associated.

For example, deficiency in a trace element provokes in turn a functional deficiency in enzymes that will then be incapable of accelerating the biochemical reactions in which they should participate. This creates a metabolic imbalance and leads to the onset of "functional" diseases. These conditions are not easy to diagnose precisely because they represent an advanced stage of metabolic imbalance. If no steps are taken to correct the deficiencies that cause them, there is a strong risk they will lead to actual diseases that might easily been avoided.

Of course, it is no easy matter to quantify deficiencies of this nature, given the minute amounts of these elements that we require for effective functioning. Certainly a blood test can determine such deficiencies, but it is also helpful to learn their characteristic symptoms and the disorders that are potentially associated with them.

Except in serious cases of deficiency, where the intervention of a trained medical professional is necessary, we can easily address minor or average deficiencies by taking a daily dose of a biocolloidal complex that is rich in all essential elements (for example, clay milk) and, in most cases, is capable of restoring balance to the body.

DEFICIENCIES WITH MULTIPLE CAUSES

It goes without saying that ideally our primary source of various nutrients, minerals, and trace elements should be our diet. But we have looked at the challenges our diet faces these days. And it is possible that other factors besides diet are involved that effect the bioavailability of the elements we do take in, such as our digestive capabilities and our ability to easily assimilate food. A deficiency can actually be linked to a number of factors, all of which need to be taken into account. As a result, it is often the case that a deficiency in one essential element cannot be satisfied simply by taking a supplement of this element alone. A blend of necessary elements may be called for in order to avoid the risk of a cascade reaction of one deficiency leading to another.

One important question must be raised before proceeding with a supplement treatment: Is the deficiency actually the result of catalytic inhibition? This is when trace elements are present in the body but are rendered useless for any number of reasons, among which may be an imbalance between some of these trace elements themselves.

Following is a short list of the principal causes for a particular trace element deficiency:

- Missing intake, connected, for example, to a depleted diet
- Poor absorption, which could be due to the condition of the digestive tract, for example, and problems with assimilation
- Problems in transport, meaning that the necessary minerals are present, but because exchanges are defective, their transport to the intended area of the body no longer occurs or occurs inadequately
- Loss of the ability to utilize certain elements, even though they are present, which is often linked to the excess presence of another element (for example, excess magnesium hinders absorption of calcium and vice versa)
- Loss of the ability to eliminate elements that hinder utilization of those we need
- Poor relationship between elements, which must often work together for proper functioning of the whole
- Unregulated exchanges, when no functions seem to be working correctly and all metabolic exchanges seem to have broken down

It is worth mentioning again several factors that are absolutely necessary to ward off mineral deficiency:

The ability to firmly affix minerals. Many of us live in a state that can be described as "clogged" because of poor dietary habits and the destructive effects of our modern lifestyle (which may include being sedentary, stressed, poorly oxygenated, or medically intoxicated). This eventually reduces our ability to firmly affix the minerals we take in. Thus, even though we are eating correctly, we are still in a depleted state—or sub-depleted state, which is to say in a state of excessive mineral loss (such as occurs with a hemorrhage of gastro-enteritis, for example) wherein the body can no longer manage to compensate for any deficiencies.

A healthy digestive tract. In order for the body to assimilate what it takes in easily, the digestive tract must be in a state of perfect operation. A prolonged period of constipation or chronic diarrhea will disrupt the absorption of minerals and trace elements. Some of these, such as iron, which must be absorbed from the duodenum, can be absorbed by the body only at specific levels in the digestive tract.

Proper proportions. The proper proportion of elements is essential. An over-abundance of one element generally leads to or signifies the deficiency of another. Taking any one specific element too often carries a risk of disrupting the balance of the whole. Proper proportions of elements will vary from one person to the next based on each individual's cellular environment.

Forms and combinations consumed. It is necessary that minerals and trace elements are present in the body in a form that it recognizes and accepts. The body will turn up its nose to cocktails of synthetic elements. Just as the body absorbs chelated and nonchelated minerals or colloidal and noncolloidal minerals differently, so does it assimilate variations of a particular element differently. For example, bivalent iron (Fer++) offers a bioavailability that is far superior to that of trivalent iron (Fer+++). In addition, to be absorbed effectively, some minerals require the presence of other minerals. Iron, for instance, requires the participation of nickel, molybdenum, and copper in order to be assimilated properly. And finally, Dr. Jacques Jane writes:

> There exist autotrophic life forms that are capable of directly assimilating mineral elements. This is not the case for animal organisms. In order to be assimilated by animals or humans, minerals must first be integrated by plants or microorganisms into organic molecules.[5]
>
> This takes us right back to our colloidal cocktails of marine or plant origin!

As we can see, mineral deficiency is a much more complex problem than it might at first seem to be, and its treatments can be just as varied and complex. If you suspect that you have a mineral deficiency, before experimenting with a free-form oligotherapy that carries the risk of doing as much harm as good, it is strongly advised that you seek the assistance of a trained specialist in this field. Remember: That trace elements are small does not mean that their effect is small, and only naturally occurring trace element complexes are free of any toxic effects.

FIRST A CHECK-UP

Before giving any prescription (at least in the event it involves a long term treatment of the internal cellular environment), a therapist will probably request a detailed balance sheet of your personal dosages in trace elements and heavy metals (which can be toxic when present in excessive amounts). There are two basic techniques to gather this information:

Blood analysis. A simple blood test can be barely sufficient—and even entirely inaccurate—when certain deficiencies are suspected. In fact, blood levels of certain elements can change from one minute to the next, depending on circumstances. For example, the fearful start we experience when crossing the street in the path of an oncoming car is enough to cause a vertiginous drop in blood calcium levels.

A blood analysis, accompanied by a plasma analysis, serves to establish a baseline profile

Hair analysis. Hair acts as a kind of accumulator of elements and can give us a reliable picture of their bioavailability at a certain time, over a period that can vary from several weeks to as long as several months (the growth of one centimeter of hair is generally equal to three to four weeks). This makes it possible to assess precisely the trace-element condition of an individual, with the understanding that a deficiency observed in one element most often corresponds to multiple deficiencies because of their interrelationships. Hair analysis can also help to determine if there are any toxic excesses of heavy metals in the body. There are a number of laboratories today that offer this kind of analysis.

AVOID EXCESS

Once you have established a blood and/or hair analysis, you should remember, before going forward, that excess can be as dangerous as a deficiency. In nutritional matters, the best advice is, "Use your common sense and avoid deficiencies and excesses with equal zeal." In the case of vitamins, minerals, and trace elements, we are programmed to receive specific amounts. When these are not met, we show signs of deficiencies; when they are exceeded—most notably in the case of trace elements—we can sometime exhibit the symptoms of being poisoned.

How do we avoid this excess? Recommendations have been made for each trace element: As a general rule, it is best never to take more than three to five times more than the recommended daily allowance and to take all supplements in intermittent treatments.

Here are some pieces of sound advice provided by Dr. Henri Picard in his book *Utilisation thérapeutique des oligo-éléments:*

> We can forget the idea that the nutritional use of trace elements is an all or nothing matter. It is utterly necessary to respect an optimum balance between trace elements, under penalty of seriously transforming enzymatic processes and subsequently, the biochemical functioning of the body's ability to synthesize.[6]

It is for this reason that we advocate, especially for those who self-medicate, the complexes that are balanced by nature itself, which can be taken simply and efficiently in the form of a natural biocolloidal water such as the Quinton's Marine Plasma products or T. J. Clark's colloidal mineral products.

14

TWO NATURAL SOURCES
OF COLLOIDAL
MINERAL COMPLEXES

T. J. CLARK: THE BURIED TREASURE
OF THE PAIUTE INDIANS

The only known colloidal minerals from plant origin come from the remnants of a primeval tropical forest in Utah.

Our story begins in Utah in 1920, on the property of a rancher suffering from kidney stones, which no known therapies of the time had been successful in treating.

After hearing their friend's complaints about his illness, the surviving elders of the Paiute tribe decided that they would bring him to a sacred spring renowned for its curative properties. Until that time they had kept this veritable fountain of youth a secret, for it dispensed water that served as the basis of their pharmacopoeia. Although doubtful of the natives' claims, the rancher eventually decided there would be no harm in testing them, so he scooped up some of the water in his hands and drank a small amount. Before leaving the site, he filled a gourd with more of the water so that he could continue the therapy, drinking the healing water in small amounts. As it happened, several weeks of this treatment were sufficient to entirely cure him of his affliction. The rancher felt free and easy in his movements, and noted, to his shock, that his kidney stones seemed to have entirely disappeared.

Once he had recovered from his initial elation, he told himself that it would not be fair to keep this "discovery" to himself and that it was absolutely imperative to allow others to benefit from it. After making several geological probes he found that this miraculous water in fact flowed beneath his own property.

He then encouraged his neighbors, who were also suffering from kidney stones, to sample the water—and everyone was amazed at the outcome. As word of the healing spring spread, people suffering from other illnesses such as digestive, joint, and circulation disorders, began collecting the water and drinking it with the same dramatic results.

Word of the waters' miraculous powers soon spread throughout the region. It was used to treat a multitude of illnesses and disorders—including such skin disorders as stubborn acne or psoriasis—with the same positive results. The fame of the spring spread into neighboring states. But alas, one day—as in the classic film *Manon of the Spring*—the miraculous water ceased to flow and its virtues became the stuff of legend, passed on by the last survivors of an era when the ground was still fertile and the waters were still pure. But is this the end of our story?

It was at this point that the rancher was struck by a brilliant notion. Having been told by several doctors that the therapeutic properties of this water were closely connected to the characteristics of the ground through which it traveled, he decided to have made a detailed geological survey of the area.

In the words of the rancher's own grandson: "The geologists discovered that the surrounding terrain contained 'pockets' of semifossilized prehistoric plants that had been miraculously preserved for approximately seventy-five to one hundred fifty million years, by the geological structure of the underground layers."

Before reemerging in a remote cave located in the tail end of the Utah mountains, this water travels through a layer of semifossilized plant matter from the Secondary (Mesozoic) Era and becomes charged with minerals and trace elements that are roughly one hundred million years old. It is clear that the Paiute Indians had at their disposal a treasure equal in value to a gold mine. It was a mine of health that was the only one of its kind, unique because it contained 72 minerals and trace elements and some twenty hyper-trace elements that have been combined over the centuries into electro-colloidal clusters (molecular polymers). As a result, the natives of Utah benefited for centuries from a natural colloidal solution directly from the ground that had the ability to treat a large number of health conditions.

THE ONLY SUCH DEPOSIT IN THE WORLD

The United States Department of the Interior has estimated the age of the unique mineral deposit beneath the Utah spring as dating from the Cretacean Era, approximately 60 million to 127 million years ago. The minerals were preserved by a chance combination of circumstances about which no precise findings have been made, though they likely followed a volcanic eruption that buried this valley beneath a fine layer of ash and mud that was neither thick nor heavy enough to crush all plant life into petroleum or coal. The climate was quite dry, which kept the plants from becoming totally fossilized or petrified so that they never transformed into rock. The deposit was then covered by a layer of sandstone some 20 to 30 feet thick, the precise amount required to protect its minerals from alteration by either high temperatures or excessive pressure. In addition, the deposit sat on top of a kind of platform of very hard clay, which allowed minerals to accumulate by preventing them from infiltrating the rock and disappearing into the soil. It has been estimated that this valuable deposit contains no less than 72 organic minerals. During the era that witnessed the formation of this reserve, dinosaurs, many of whom weighed more than 70 tons, inhabited the earth. Perhaps their impressive size could be reasonably ascribed to the extremely mineral rich plant life that formed their essential diet?

Today, the remnants of this prehistoric tropical forest have become an underground mine, and its plant-derived minerals, preserved in their primary state, are steeped in water in accordance with a specific procedure that determines their concentration. A complex system of filtration ensures that the liquid contains only organic colloidal minerals. What is obtained at the spring, therefore, is a mix of minerals and elements in a form that the body can assimilate perfectly without the addition of any chemical products. Nor does this water require preservatives or irradiation; it preserves itself naturally. This concentrated solution was analyzed by the German doctor Fritz-Albert Popp, a nominee for the Nobel Prize in biophysics. His tests revealed that those colloidal minerals originating in prehistoric plant life increased the cellular output of vital (electric) energy far beyond the optimal limits that had been established earlier.

A JOB FOR SPECIALISTS

Because water no longer circulates through these geological layers naturally, the mineral transfer must now take place in the laboratory with water from another spring that has been filtered through blocks of fossilized plant matter extracted from Cretacean layers some 200 feet beneath the earth. This particular spring has only recently come back to life.

Today, this mineral deposit is regarded as the only one of its kind on the planet. Digging the fossilized plant matter in this valley could be described as making hay—though the hay is 100 million years old! Semi-fossilized blades of grass, leaves, needles, pinecones, and bark can all be recognized in the overturned soil.

Harvesting from this deposit is entrusted to highly skilled miners. They must find a way to penetrate the earth far below the surface, the sole place where this exceptional and unique mineral compound can be extracted, and bring it back up to the surface. Although they have the most modern equipment available to assist them, they employ only natural methods to remove these minerals. Once they have been prepared, they are "filtered" from the ore just as they would be by nature: through a current of fresh, pure water.

The colloidal water intended to serve as the support for this mineral cocktail is prepared as follows: The plant debris is reduced to a fine powder, one that is quite similar to high quality white flour. This powder is then steeped for three to four weeks in filtered spring water; when it has reached the specific gravity of 3.0, which is quite heavy, it contains 38 grams of colloidal minerals per liter. This specific product has been available commercially since 1926. It is the only nutritional product to have ever received a legal consent decree from a federal court and the approval of the U.S. Department of Health and Human Services to be packaged and sold as a nutritional supplement. It is currently marketed as T. J. Clark's Colloidal Minerals.

A TRUE PANACEA

A number of health conditions have been successfully treated with this mineral-rich water. Its pH is 3.2 and because its trace elements come from fossilized plant matter, it is especially anionic, or electronegative.

Dr. Jean-Pierre Willem describes it thus:

> Biocolloidal water has the property of completely covering our diseased or damaged cells and restoring them to their full capacity. This water, which is also known as biocatalyzed or vitalized water, heals and repairs lesions, accelerates the rate of plant growth and immunizes plants against parasites and illnesses, and restores the electromagnetic structures of the cells and ensures the balanced frequency of their oscillations, an essential condition for cellular life.

Recent research has emphasized these characteristics. In fact, as this water passes through and emerges from the semi-fossilized plant matter untainted by pollutants, it breaks off pieces of plant fossils whose trace elements are primarily anionic and electronegative. These highly energetic microparticles remain suspended in the water in a colloidal form.

The absence of electrons spells the thermodynamic death of the human machine that can no longer metabolize nutrients. Ironically, we are all living in an industrial civilization that is impoverishing the electrical terrain of our body. Our depleted bodies on alkaline and oxidized land lack the negative electrons necessary to assure proper metabolic reactions. Oxidants like the chlorine and ozone in our sterilized waters, vaccines, chemical medications, and free radicals, are all greedy for electrons. They are ceaselessly capturing them, thereby impoverishing the physical electrical environment and gradually depriving our body of its metabolic capabilities.

This water's extremely stable microparticles (with their strong electronegative field determined by the electronegative potential of electrons) contain minerals that are capable of energizing virtually all other nutrients they encounter.[1]

In his annual report, Dr. LaFave of the U.S. Metabolic Research Center, added this commentary: "By providing the cells some 72 trace elements in a form that can be directly and easily assimilated, T. J. Clark's colloidal solution deeply 'cleanses' the cells and restores the body's mineral balance in spectacular fashion."

Dr. Michael Zimmerman, the head of the department in a clinic specializing in the treatment of chronic illnesses that have resisted conventional treatments, has added his confirmation of the above statement with this remark made at the conclusion of clinical tests:

> The human body requires the complete range of trace elements ideally available in nature. These substances are the basic building blocks for the living world. The assimilation of vitamins and amino acids and the production of enzymes and hormones depend entirely on this daily intake of trace elements, the doses of which are infinitesimal in size, yet these minerals are by and large absent from our deficient diets.

Interestingly, Linus Pauling (winner of the Nobel Prize for his work in molecular chemistry and of the Nobel Peace Prize) regularly imbibed this therapeutic water and became one of its staunchest advocates.

The natural richness of colloidal trace elements in T. J. Clark's water matches almost exactly the ideal balance[2] and inspired the following commentary from Dr. Jean-Pierre Willem:

> Researchers have thus discovered that these stable and practically indestructible micells contribute a significant amount of electricity to human metabolism in particular. They allow for the maintenance of cellular life and, most important, for the retriggering of physicochemical or enzymatic reactions that have ceased. They reactivate all the fluid in the body, making it highly energized. I am no longer at all surprised to see that T. J. Clark's solution has restored life to infected or deteriorated tissue.

The pathologies that this colloidal solution of trace elements and minerals affects are obviously quite numerous, given that all the elements it contains have a role to play in the regulation of the internal cellular environment of the body.

What works for human beings will also work for animals. Our animal companions are also suffering from mineral depletion and can likewise benefit from a colloidal solution of trace elements and minerals, whether they drink it or have it applied as a lotion.

QUINTON'S MARINE PLASMA: SEAWATER WITH HEALING PROPERTIES

The French physiologist and biologist René Quinton (1866–1925) is one of the many researchers who, though obscure today, enjoyed great notoriety and wide regard in his lifetime. His research focused primarily on the therapeutic values of seawater—in fact, at the beginning of the twentieth century his discovery of its remarkable properties made it possible for him to save countless people (and animals) from serious, life- threatening illnesses such as gastroenteritis, children's cholera, and tuberculosis.

René Quinton's work logically led him to his greatest discovery: the resemblance between seawater—from which all life emerged—and that of our internal cellular environment, which he described as "the water of our aquarium." The sole difference between the two is that while the concentration of seawater borders on 33 grams of total salts per liter, that of our internal cellular environment is only 9 grams a liter.

THE NUTRITIVE ELEMENTS OF SEAWATER

The sea holds the basic characteristics of everything that exists on the earth. It contains all the minerals and trace elements that are necessary for all living cells. Gregory and Ovenberger have shown that the marine saline matrix contains all 92 elements listed on the Periodic Table.

Seawater is an environment of extraordinary diversity and complexity whose mysteries are far from all being solved. The elements that make up the marine saline matrix present specific properties that cannot explain its composition on their own. For example, differences have been observed between the properties of seawater with 33 percent salinity and an equivalent solution of sea salts dissolved again in distilled water. The coefficient of the dissociation of the salts present in the seawater is higher than that observed in the solution with a distilled water base and, contrary to what occurs in a "reconstituted" solution, the majority of the constituent elements of seawater are never saturated, despite their higher concentration.

It has also been observed that although the total saline concentration of seawater may vary, its relative concentration of different ions remains almost constant (Dittmar's Law). This is what gives Quinton's

Marine Plasma—which, unlike reconstituted and treated seawater products, is entirely natural—its full value.

FROM THE VORTEX TO SPECIFIC PROPERTIES

Based on earlier test readings, René Quinton had determined certain zones where he could find pure living water to be used as samples for the preparation of his "plasma." The water that is used today to make Quinton's Marine Plasma is still taken from these same zones. They are referred to technically as vortexes and display swirling currents, a constant temperature, and an unvarying (or only slightly varying) mineral composition, which is why the phytoplankton and zooplankton that reproduce there are so stable. Collected from depths of 100 feet and 30 feet above the ocean floor, the water is analyzed and filtered on site, then transported to laboratories under controlled conditions at a temperature that is kept at 4 degrees Celsius inside a special chamber for a maximum of 45 days.

The seawater is then sterilized through a microfiltration process of 0.22 micron performed in cold temperatures with a microporous filter (the water is never heated). Finally, the water is sealed in vials. The fruits of this effort are a natural seawater with a ratio of 30 to 35 grams of salt per liter.*

Of course, it is necessary to match this seawater to the isotonic fluid of the cellular enviroment by adding some nonmineral spring water. As during Quinton's time—when the seawater was diluted with natural spring water—the water today is mixed with heated, distilled water that lends its diluting properties to the product. This results in a concentration of 9 grams of salt per liter, the original Quinton's Marine Plasma.†
"Seawater is a living environment that displays a remarkable mineral balance in comparison to that of the body. All of its elements occur naturally in sizes and proportions quite close to those encountered in the internal cellular environment of the body, and form a very active biological synergy."[3]

---

*Currently sold as Quinton's Drinkable Hypertonic.

†Now sold under the name of Quinton's Drinkable Isotonic.

HUMAN PLASMA AND SEAWATER

The bioavailability of the trace elements contained in seawater in a natural and balanced complete ionic diffusion makes it possible to avoid the problems of assimilation and absorption that come with elements in other forms. Most important is that the minerals and trace elements in this seawater are in a concentration that is quite close to that of the body's internal cellular environment. René Quinton's twenty-five years of work with his medical team made it possible for him to understand both the therapeutic applications of precisely prepared seawater and the influence it could have on the ionic and mineral equilibrium of the body.

THE THERAPEUTIC VIRTUES OF QUINTON'S MARINE PLASMA

Just like the "prehistoric water" discussed in chapter 13, seawater provides a veritable cocktail of trace elements to which we can attribute its many therapeutic properties. The simple addition of this seawater to a daily diet has brought about improvement in if not outright cures of all kinds of disorders and diseases.

Regulation of the pH

Because its pH falls between 7.9 and 8.3, seawater offers a significant buffering power, an important factor to those whose bodies are suffering from an overly acidified internal environment. Especially noteworthy, however, is seawater's regulatory effect. Not only will a hydromarine cure rectify the problem of over-acidification, it will have the same effect on an internal cellular environment that is overly alkaline. By itself, this regulating ability goes a long way toward explaining the therapeutic results of marine cures, for the regeneration of the body's internal cellular environment encourages the elimination of toxins from the body.

A Powerful Regulating and Regenerating Effect

Research performed by scientists including Jarricot, Hansche, and Bensch has demonstrated the powerful regenerating and regulating effect of this marine plasma, which acts to return equilibrium to the potassium, sodium, and magnesium ions that are essential to the proper functioning of the nervous system.

Due to its unique electrolytic composition, seawater also possesses a powerful regulating action on gastric and intestinal pH. For this reason it can be effective in combating all kinds of digestive disorders. It can likewise be used to treat all types of allergies efficiently. As Bensch offers: "It fundamentally modifies the mineral content of different tissues by correcting ionic imbalances, which explains the favorable effect it has on allergic diseases. In clinical settings both the subjective and objective results were so favorable that it gave the impression of a specific curative effect."[4]

Concerning magnesium, the importance of which inspired Norris to describe it as "the essential cation," after fourteen patients received three weeks of treatment consisting of 250 cc of seawater daily, blood magnesium levels were observed to be eight to ten times higher than before treatment.

Another positive effect was noted in Dr. Jarricot's research: Following a perfusion (the passage of fluid through tissue) of Quinton's Marine Plasma, the kidneys eliminated twice the volume of urine (in both liquid and solid particles) than they did following a perfusion of a synthetic physiological serum.

In another study, Rompler treated thirty cases of gastritis caused by food allergies with 250 cc of seawater taken twice daily for a period of three weeks. Among the results he observed were:

- A gradual increase in bilirubin
- An increase in trypasin
- An increase in intestinal enzymes
- Normalization of gastric acid levels
- Disappearance of the usual clinical symptoms exhibited in such cases (flatulence, intestinal meteorism, heartburn, digestive difficulties).

Other positive effects of marine plasma have been noted. The work of Eppinger and Hess has shown that the assimilation of seawater taken orally is much slower than the assimilation of freshwater and that it performs an important regulatory function on the balance of the cations of potassium, sodium, magnesium, and cacium, all of which are necessary for proper functioning of the nervous system. The research of Kaufer and Keining points to a finding that bronchial asthma manifests in an internal environment whose nervous system is unstable, a circumstance that is aggravated by electrolytic imbalance. This finding seemed to be confirmed by the treatment of fourteen asthmatics with Quinton's Marine Plasma, which resulted in immediate improvement for two of the patients and revealed tangible results for all after one to three weeks.

Quinton's Marine Plasma, which can be taken orally or by subcutaneous injection, offers therapeutic effects for the following conditions:

- Mental and physical fatigue, which are often linked to a mineral imbalance, as are memory problems, difficulties with concentrating and sleeping, spasmophilia, irritability, and stress.
- Digestive disorders, such as hepatobiliary problems, stomach disorders, colitis, diarrhea, constipation, and diseases of the aerodigestive tract (gastritis, colic, etc.), which are often connected to a disruption in the body's acid-alkaline balance. Treatments with seawater base have led to improvement in the condition of the mucous membrane of the entire digestive tract. Quinton and Jarricot used seawater to successfully treat numerous cases of enteritis and disorders that involved the inability to assimilate food accompanied by stubborn constipation or excessive diarrhea. In addition, it had the positive effect of regulating the body's fluids, thereby addressing dehydration and the regulation of the large intestine.
- Allergies and allergic processes of all kinds. The work of Bensch, based on 500 cases of allergy sufferers who were treated with oral doses of seawater revealed improvements in all cases.
- Skin Disorders, which are often the result of digestive disorders or allergies, and thus are related to the availability of trace elements and the regulation of pH in the blood and in the skin. Using marine plasma therapeutically, Quinton obtained excellent results with cases of psoriasis, eczema, various mycoses, and all afflictions of the skin and phaneres that are due to high acidity.
- Circulatory problems, which marine plasma addresses by regulating the blood pH and the body's fluids, and increasing the flow of blood when it is overcharged with toxins. In the case of

high blood pressure, Quinton's Marine Plasma is still indicated, despite its high sodium chloride content. Research has shown that most important is supplying the body with all the trace elements and minerals it needs (which includes calcium) and that a regulatory effect is often a natural consequence of satisfying these physical requirements. Of course, in the case of those who are on a strict salt-free diet, a doctor's supervision is definitely called for.

- Immune system support against infections, which, as Béchamp points out, have more to do with the internal cellular environment than with external microbes. Much like colloidal trace elements, seawater, with its trace elements such as copper, manganese, and magnesium, has a positive effect on the thymus, which leads to boosting the immune system. Quinton obtained remarkable results using seawater to address lowered immune system response and infection in babies and young children. His plasma worked wonders in cases of diarrhea and dehydration. As a preventive measure, pregnant women are advised to drink a vial of marine plasma once a day for the first six months of their pregnancy, then to continue using this supplement throughout the entire time they are nursing their children, which helps to ensure that the baby's immune system matures to its optimum potential.

- Hemorrhages and blood loss, which seawater addresses through the rapid restoration of proper hemoglobin levels. There has been ample demonstration that a perfusion of marine plasma can take the place of blood transfusions with none of the risks that transfusions may incur. In these cases, proper hemoglobin levels are rapidly restored and phagocytosis is greatly improved.

The original marine therapy of René Quinton was first made available in 1904 in a form that could be either taken orally or injected. In France, Quinton's Marine Plasma in a form for intravenous or subcutaneous use has not been authorized to be sold commercially since 1984. Laws passed at that time required all injectable products to be sterilized at high temperatures, which would render Quinton's Marine Plasma virtually ineffective by essentially causing the loss of its trace elements.

It is still possible, however, to read in the old Vidal dictionary* about some of the therapeutic effects of seawater taken intravenously. These include:

- A regenerative effect brought about by the replacement of an internal cellular environment that has been depleted or polluted
- A rebalancing of minerals
- A recharging of trace elements resulting in the creation of trace synergies (catalysts)
- Homeopathic activity of certain elements

In fact, through bioavailability, "seawater behaves like a natural reservoir of cellular micronutrients, a veritable manna for regulating the surrounding tissue, which finds itself literally drowned in this miniature primordial bath of life. Whole capillary networks are immediately swollen with this liquid. According to Doctor Salmanoff, author of *Secrets et sagesse du corps,* the output of the capillaries can increase by as much as 700 percent. With such massive rehydration, the process of decay is halted and can even be reversed."[5]

QUINTON'S MARINE PLASMA AND T. J. CLARK'S COLLOIDAL MINERALS: UNIQUE MODES OF TREATMENT

As Dr. Jarricot puts it, "Marine plasma is not a serum to be used against this or that affliction; it is for the *living cell.*" The diversity of the indications of these natural colloidal solutions only more deeply emphasizes their activity: targeting by their very nature the restoration of health, no matter what disorder is involved.

Like the Utah spring and the product manufactured from it, seawater is a natural colloidal solution and the primordial source of the trace elements present in our cells. The great advantage of both is that they are very easy to assimilate and contain all the trace elements the body uses in the amounts corresponding to the equilibrium of the body's internal cellular environment. Their interactions with the body open a field of

---

*A standard French drug reference.

research that is almost limitless, and we are surely only beginning to learn what they can offer. The research that has been performed to date has already shown their effectiveness and versatility, indicating an important role for them in preventive medicine. They are remarkable natural remedies for our bodies that have become either imbalanced or plainly depleted through today's lifestyle and diet choices.

A SHORT HANDBOOK
OF OLIGOTHERAPY FOR
TRACE ELEMENTS

Perhaps you still harbor some doubts about the real necessity of minerals and trace elements? Or perhaps you have read about them before this, or have even taken them on occasion, but without a very clear idea of what they are or what purpose they truly serve. The best solution might be to present some specific examples of the therapeutic properties attributed to them.

Of course, the study of trace elements in the body must take into account the multiple interactions that are at play there. Not all researchers are in agreement on the properties that are attributed to these elements. It is easy to see that researching the precise action of an element taken on its own is no easy task. Some of the factors to consider in the results are the form of the trace element taken, the subject's internal cellular environment, and the presence or deficiency of certain other elements. No element can be studied outside its overall context. While everyone is in agreement on some of the properties of the essential trace elements, there is no unanimity on those properties attributed to lesser-known electrolytes. It is important that we all be aware of this.

Here we will take an overview of the essential positive properties, therapeutic effects, and possible interactions of fifty-three trace elements. While the virtues of some of these substances are now fairly well-known, there are others over which opinions differ, and some whose precise properties remain unknown but whose presence is still essential in the overall functioning of our bodies. All of them are considered in their trace element and colloidal form (as discussed earlier, their properties will not always be similar to that of their mineral counterparts taken in a measurable form).

It should be noted that some of these trace elements are not available in all countries—at least not in single, separate units. On the other hand, all of them can be found in complex formulas. Some dietary supplements also add this complete range of trace elements to their mineral complexes. For example, the American company Nature's Plus has created a formulation containing 72 trace elements from "primordial seawater" that have been naturally chelated with marine sediments from very deep waters, which support a chelated mineral complex in the exact proportions existing in this primordial seawater.*

Warning: We are discussing only **trace elements** here! While minerals and metals are not at all toxic taken in the form of trace elements, some minerals and metals are **extremely toxic** when taken in measurable doses.

Aluminum (Al)
Indicated for insomnia, memory problems, and mental disorders
Aluminum in colloidal form is one of the elements found in abundance in soil and plants. It is a trace element that has a significant presence in the brain, whose functioning it appears to regulate. A substance with a transformational effect on the body's internal cellular environment, a deficiency of this mineral is generally betrayed by difficulties in concentration and memorization, slow learning, a state of nervousness, and insomnia. It also acts as an inhibitor of certain enzymes. Its level in the body is about 1 mg per kg in most tissue. Aluminum is an essential element of human nutrition in its colloidal form. It forms an important combination with lithium.

---

*These are sold under the names of Trace-Mins, Ultra-Mins, Ultra-Two Light, Mega Force, Mini-Plex, and Mini Mins.

Indicated for use in the treatment of:
- Minor insomnia in adults and children older than six years
- Atony of all kinds, including cerebral
- Memory difficulties in the elderly
- Intellectual deficiencies and mental disorders
- Slow intellectual development in children with Downs Syndrome
- Aftereffects of vaccinal encephalitis
- Children's minor problems adapting to school

Antimony (Sb)

Indicated for arthritis and chronic illnesses

Antimony is a biocatalyst for arthritic internal cellular environments and those displaying a tendency toward chronic illness.

Indicated for use in the treatment of:
- Osteoarthritis, arthritis
- Bronchitis, chronic head colds
- Chronic hepatitis
- Prostate problems
- Acute rheumatism

Arsenic (As)

Indicated for support of immune system defenses

This trace element is present in all life forms. It has no toxic properties when in its colloidal form. A hyper-trace, it is generally present in mammals at a level of 0.07 to 0.2 mg per kg. Daily we need 0.01 to 0.03 mg of Arsenic.

Specific properties:
- Improves internal cellular environment
- Supports the body's immune defenses
- Plays a role in phosphorylation, a stage in the transformation of glucose into glycogen
- Maintains health of bones, teeth, and hair

Indicated for use in the treatment of:
- Chronic bronchitis, asthma, pulmonary emphysema, tuberculosis
- Grippe, angina, and respiratory disorders
- Ganglional problems, intestinal disorders

- Bone and joint problems
- Anemia, convalescence, overexertion
- Depressed appetite
- Depression, neurasthenia (rebuilds nerve cells)

Barium (Ba)

Indicated for biocatalysis

Though we do not fully understand its role, barium is a transformative agent on the internal cellular environment. It is known to play a role as a biocatalyst in a number of physical processes.

Indicated for use in the treatment of:
- Senescence
- High blood pressure

Bismuth (Bi)

Indicated for angina, sore throats

Bismuth alters the internal cellular environment of infectious states in the ORL sphere and for grippe. A bismuth-lead-tin combination is used in the treatment of syphilis and cancer.

Specific Properties:
- Acts as an anti-infectant
- Supports the body's immune system

Indicated for use in the treatment of:
- Angina, laryngitis, amygdalitis
- Gastric and duodenal ulcers
- Syphilis
- Cancer

Boron (B)

Indicated for effective calcium absorption

Boron is a hyper-trace element present in soil and plants, which contain much more of it than animals. We normally have about 0.01 mg of boron per kg of body weight. Breast milk contains a higher amount, averaging 0.08 mg per liter. Boron specifically affixes to the liver, kidneys, bones, and central nervous system. It is toxic in large doses.

Specific Properties:
- Plays a role in bone and muscle development
- Stimulates cerebral function and mental alertness
- Plays a role in metabolizing calcium, phosphorus, copper, magnesium, and vitamin D and in the fixation of calcium
- Plays a role in the secretion of estrogen and testosterone

Indicated for use in the treatment of:
- Osteoporosis
- Menopause difficulties
- Contraindicated in cases of rheumatoid arthritis

Bromium (Br)

Indicated for soothing of the nervous system

Bromium is another hyper-trace element. Blood plasma contains 1 atom of bromium for every 1,700 atoms of chloride. It is found in the bodies of humans and higher mammals at about 0.1 mg per kg. Bromium settles primarily in the pituitary gland.

Specific Properties:
- Plays a role in membranous exchanges
- Acts as a sedative on the nervous system

Cadmium (Cd)

Cadmium is a hyper-trace element whose specific properties remain a mystery, though we know it is present in the body and that it take part in various metabolic exchanges. In case of overdose, cadmium's antidote is copper.

Calcium (Ca)

Indicated for health of the bones, teeth, and nervous system

An adult requires a daily intake of about 900 mg of this basic mineral, though pregnant or menopausal women, adolescents, and those over age 65 need as much as 1 gram or more daily. Calcium deficiency is revealed by various problems ranging from the appearance of dental cavities to osteoporosis, decalcification, childhood rickets, muscle cramps, spasmophilia, nervousness, sleep problems, kidney stones, and disorders causing subcutaneous loss of pigmentation. Be forewarned that taking excessive amounts of calcium can be detrimental to health.

Taking more than 2 grams per day greatly increases the risk of developing hypercalcimia (excessive calcium in the blood) accompanied by constipation, arterial high blood pressure, and nausea. Here again, taking it in a colloidal form avoids any risk of an overdose and enables it to act more selectively on the nervous system.

Don't believe for an instant that you consume enough dairy products to supply all your body's calcium needs. In reality, eating large quantities of dairy foods can actually lead to decalcification (for more on this see page 18 in chapter 2). It is important to note that calcium cannot be assimilated properly without the supporting presence of other trace elements

Specific Properties:
- Encourages growth and maintains health of bones and teeth
- Plays a role in increasing bone mass (especially in children and menopausal women)
- Plays a role in muscular development
- Maintains gum health
- Plays a role in the prevention of kidney stones
- Maintains balance in the nervous system
- Regularizes heart rate, arrythmia, tachycardia
- Regularizes nerve impulse transmission
- Regularizes blood coagulation
- Regularizes blood pressure
- Plays a role in the prevention of cancer (especially colorectal cancer)
- Regularizes cholesterol
- Plays a role in the prevention of cardiovascular disease
- Plays a role in the prevention of eclampsia in pregnant women
- Plays a role in metabolizing of numerous vitamins
- Maintains permeability of the cell membrane
- Regulates blood pH (when taken in measurable amounts)
- Plays a role in preventing the assimilation of lead and its deposit in the teeth and bones

Indicated for use in the treatment of:
- Sprains, lumbago
- Muscle cramps, contractions
- Tetany, spasmophilia

- Headaches
- Tingling and stinging sensations, numbness
- Insomnia, depression
- Anxiety, aggressiveness
- Varicose veins, hemorrhoids
- Biliary atonia
- Visceral ptosis
- Fibroids
- Pregnancy (promotes calcification of baby's bones, prevents maternal bone loss, promotes strong muscular contraction), nursing (promotes high quality milk)
- Eczema, rashes, fistula, abscesses

Carbon (C)

Indicated for digestive tract health

Carbon, the very foundation of organic chemistry, is the fundamental building block of living matter whose formation, evolution, and decay forms what is called the carbon cycle. Its effectiveness against digestive disorders when taken in measurable amounts is well known. As a trace element it is an essential catalyst.

Specific Properties:

- Plays a role in intracellular exchanges
- Balances humoral fluids
- Supports the body's immune system
- Acts as an anti-infectant (especially in the digestive tract)

Indicated for use in the treatment of:

- Left-side enterocolitis (according to Ménétrier)
- Hepatic insufficiencies

Cerium (Ce)

Cerium is a hyper-trace element in the body that acts as a biocatalyst. Some believe it to be helpful against eye and vision problems.

Cesium (Cs)

Indicated for biocatalysis

Cesium is a biocatalyst and an agent of change in the body's internal cellular environment. Our body, like that of all vertebrates, contains on average 32 mg per kg of body weight.

Specific Properties:
- Supports the body's immune system
- Regulates cardiac rhythm

Chloride (C)
Indicated for Cardiac rhythm
Interestingly, in blood plasma, 8 atoms of selenium can be counted for every million chloride atoms. The electrolytic function of chloride makes it crucial to the proper functioning of the "body electric."

Specific Properties:
- Governs intra- and extra-cellular balance

Indicated for use in the treatment of:
- Muscle weakness
- Disturbed heart rhythm (i.e., arythmia or tachycardia)
- Chronic fatigue

Chromium (Cr)
Indicated for regulation of glycemia
We require only a small allowance of this mineral, on the order of 50 to 200 mcg (micrograms). Diabetics, athletes, and people taking diuretics need a higher intake—no less than 200 mcg daily. It seems that the amount of chromium in the body diminishes with age. Like zinc, it seems to play a role in the spatial structure of DNA. Its strongest concentrations are found in the liver, spleen, ovaries, testicles, lymphocytes, and bones.

Specific properties:
- Plays a role in metabolizing glucose
- Acts as an insulin cofactor
- Acts to improve glucose tolerance
- Acts to retrigger vital energy
- Regularizes blood cholesterol (encourages HDL, the good cholesterol)
- Plays a role in the prevention of cardiovascular disease (chromium deficiency often signals coronary problems)
- Plays a role in the synthesis of proteins

- Acts as a hypotensive
- Encourages the growth of lean muscle tissue over fat

Indicated for use in the treatment of:
- Glycemia, diabetes (even insulin-dependant diabetes), and hypoglycemia
- Anxiety or fatigue

Cobalt (Co)

Indicated for migraines

Cobalt is present in the body only as a trace element. It is one of the constituents of vitamin B_{12}, which contains 4 percent cobalt, and aids in the formation of red blood cells. It also regulates the cerebral torus and aids circulation in this region. Although 1/10 mcg daily (most often in the form of B_{12}) is generally considered sufficient, a deficiency in this element may be the source of anemia, circulatory disorders, and migraines. Cobalt-manganese-copper is an effective combination, as is cobalt-copper-nickel.

Specific properties:
- Maintains nervous tissue
- Acts as a vasodilator
- Acts as a hypotensive
- Acts as an antispasmodic
- Plays a role in activating certain enzymes
- Activates some of the B vitamins
- Plays a role in building vitamin B_{12}, which is necessary for cellular division and synthesis of hemoglobin

Indicated for use in the treatment of:
- Difficulties affecting the sympathetic and parasympathetic nervous systems
- Hiccups
- Digestive disorders
- Migraines
- Hypoglycemia
- Arteritis, "dead finger" sensation, circulatory spasms
- Anemia (encourages the formation of red blood cells)
- Arteritis of the lower limbs
- Tachycardia

Copper (Cu)

Indicated for use as an anti-infectant and anti-inflammatory

Copper can be found in all organic tissue. An essential trace element for the body, copper takes part in complex enzymatic reactions that protect our cells from the attacks of free radicals. It is known to have hundreds of functions. Copper possesses a remarkable anti-inflammatory ability, especially against joint or rheumatoid pain. It plays a role in the synthesis of hemoglobin and the construction of bone and is an important constituent of elastic tissue. The first signs of its deficiency include gray hair, the appearance of wrinkles, varicose veins, and a loosening of the skin. Copper is also a recognized anti-infectant; it can lessen the severity of winter's infectious illnesses. The body contains 100 to 150 mg of copper, primarily in the liver, kidneys, and central nervous system. The daily requirement for an adult supplied by food and supplements is between 1.5 and 5 mg. Irrational over consumption of this element can result in poisoning.

Effective combinations include copper-gold-silver, copper-manganese, copper-cobalt, copper-nickel-cobalt, and copper-iron-manganese (which works especially well in the treatment of weight loss, preventing fatigue, irritability, and somnolence).

In the case of overdose, copper's antidote is zinc.

Specific properties:

- Acts as an antioxidant
- Like lead and zinc, acts as an enzyme inhibitor
- Supports the immune system's resistance to infections
- Plays a role in the prevention of vascular and cerebral difficulties
- Plays a role in the prevention of aneurisms
- Powerfully supports the immune system
- Protects against microbial toxins
- Activates metabolism
- Metabolizes iron
- Acts in the formation of hemoglobin and the multiplication of red cells
- Forms part of one of the basic constituents of SOD (superoxyde dismutase), the enzyme responsible for maintaining cardiac muscle tone and cellular regeneration

- Plays a role in hair and skin coloration by converting tyrosine (an amino acid) into melanin
- Accelerates the oxidation of vitamin C
- Plays a role in the synthesis of numerous enzymes (such as SOD and tyrosine) and certain hormones
- Plays a role in the prevention of sterility
- Plays a role in bone growth and the building of hemoglobin
- Increases elastin production and the formation of collagen (especially when combined with zinc and vitamin C)
- Prevents wrinkles and loose skin
- Prevents premature white hair
- Plays a role in maintaining the sense of taste
- Maintains joint health and nervous system balance
- Acts as a healing agent

Indicated for use in the treatment of:
- Infectious and viral states; viruses (grippe and its complications)
- Chronic infectious diseases
- Chronic diarrhea
- Asthenia, anorexia, anemia
- Rheumatoid cardiopthies, arteriosclerosis
- Inflammatory rheumatoid afflictions (developing chronic polyarthritis, acute articular rheumatism, ankylosing spondylarthritis)
- Pigmentation problems such as vitiligo
- Benign prostate disorders

Europium (Eu)

Europium is a rare earth. No studies have yet been conducted to determine its effect on humans, though its administration in very low doses (smaller, even, than that of trace elements) on laboratory animals seems to double their life expectancy.

Fluorine (Fl)

Indicated for strengthening of teeth and bones

Fluorine fixes calcium in the bones and to tooth enamel. It therefore plays a role in bone growth and contributes to the solidity of the skeletal structure. It also can alter the internal cellular environment of the body. Fluorine is required only in very small amounts (1 to 2 mg for adults). Amounts higher than this are harmful and carry a risk of making the bones too fragile or too dense or of imparting a characteristic pigmentation of the teeth known as fluorosis. Ideally, fluorine should be taken as a component of naturally mineralized water, where it is in balance with all other colloidal trace elements.

Specific properties:
- Prevents dental cavities, strengthens bones, and remineralizes the surface of teeth covered with dental plaque
- Plays a role in metabolizing calcium

Indicated in for use in the treatment of:
- Bone afflictions, osteoporosis, rickets
- Scoliosis, kyphosis (curvature of the spine)
- Paget's Disease
- Scheuerman's Disease
- Ligamentary hyperlaxity, any minor ligamentary affliction
- Fractures, decalcification, rheumatism, spasmophilia

Gallium (Ga)

While Gallium is present in the body, its amount and precise role remain a mystery. It is sometimes recommended in the treatment of tuberculosis.

Germanium (Ge)

Indicated for increased cellular oxygenation

A hyper-trace element, Germanium seems to play an important role in the prevention of cancer and control of the aging process. Japanese researcher Kazuhiki Asai asserts that taken in a measurable dose of 100 to 300 mg daily, Germanium would be effective in the treatment of rheumatoid polyarthritis, hypercholesterolemia, candidiasis, chronic viral infections, cancer, and AIDS.

Specific properties:
- Improves cellular oxygenation
- Supports the body's immune system
- Eliminates toxins from the body
- Acts as an analgesic

Indicated for use in the treatment of:
- Rheumatoid polyarthritis
- Hypercholesterolemia
- Candidiasis
- Chronic viral infections
- Cancer
- AIDS

Gold (Au)

Indicated for stimulation of the body's natural defenses

Gold, which presents no danger of toxicity, stimulates cellular activity. Another powerful fighter of infection, it is often combined with copper and silver. Its biological polyvalence allows it to act on all physical functions, internal cellular terrain, and organs to address whatever disease or disorder may be involved. It affixes itself primarily to the bone marrow, liver and spleen. A common effective combination is gold-copper-silver.

Specific properties:
- Stimulates cellular activity and the body's defenses
- Acts as an antitoxin
- Plays a role in the healing process of wounds
- Supports the cardiovascular system
- Acts as an anticarcinogen (especially when combined with selenium, platinum, uranium, copper, and nickel)

Indicated for use in the treatment of:
- Infectious diseases such as measles, scarlet fever, meningitis, typhus, and septicemia
- Fever
- Rheumatoid inflammation
- High blood pressure

Iodine (I)

Indicated for maintenance of thyroid and cerebral functions

Iodine deficiency is a major problem in modern societies, affecting some 20 million Europeans and 8 million people worldwide, with the greatest number of those living in Africa and Asia. Rates of iodine deficiency in the United States have quadrupled since 1976, when it affected some 2.6 percent of the population. To address this, iodine was added to salt commercially (to create the iodized salt commonly found in grocery stores today). Our bodies contain 30 to 50 mg of iodine, of which 10 to 20mg are found in the thyroid gland or, more specifically, in the hormones this gland manufactures. These hormones are dispersed throughout our bodies where they act on a cellular level to promote development and growth. Iodine deficiency can thus retard metabolism, growth, and the cerebral development of very young children. It is easy to see the importance of ensuring a proper intake of iodine, especially for pregnant women at the time of the euthyroidal development of the fetus. A baby suffering from iodine deficiency may have a retarded growth rate both mentally and physically. Nursing mothers and adolescents must also receive an adequate amount of iodine. Average adult needs are estimated to be 0.2 mg or slightly less per day.

Specific properties:
- Plays an important role in the functioning of the thyroid by acting in the synthesis of thyroidial hormones
- Regulates the thyroid
- Increases basic metabolism and all metabolic exchanges
- Plays a role in physical and mental development (iodine deficiency in infants can lead to mental retardation)
- Acts to slow aging
- Plays a role in regulating internal body temperature, the cardiovascular system, and respiratory functions
- Promotes healthy skin, nails, and hair
- Aids in metabolizing fats

Indicated for use in the treatment of:
- Conditions of thyroid imbalance: hyperthyroidism, nervosity, hypothyroidism, goiter, hyperemotionality, fatigue, obesity, or poor mental functioning linked to hypothyroidism
- Lymphatism or slow growth
- Mastitis, breast cysts
- High or low blood pressure
- Lowered fertility, false labor
- Organic sclerosis

Iron (Fe)

Indicated for anemia

Falling somewhere in between minerals and trace elements because of its presence in more significant amounts, iron is indispensable for life, despite its real toxicity when it becomes deposited in the tissue. It plays a role in multiple chemical reactions, principal of which is the transport of oxygen by hemoglobin. It is also essential to maintaining a strong immune system. Quantitatively speaking, iron is the most important trace element in our system, with its amount equaling from 3 to 5 g. Three fourths of this is found in our billions of red blood cells. Iron is also abundantly present in the liver and spleen, where it is utilized in the manufacture of new red blood cells. A deficiency in iron (originating from blood loss due to menstruation or hemorrhage, pregnancy, nursing, or periods of growth in childhood or adolescence) leads to great fatigue due to lack of cellular oxygenation. Our daily diet should supply in the neighborhood of 10 to 18 mg of iron. As a colloidal trace element, its presence alone allows the body to synthesize it naturally with no danger of a deficiency or excess.

Note: An iron deficiency is often due to either an insufficient amount of this element in the diet or blood loss, but it could also be due to a deficiency of vitamin B_6 or B_{12}. Although the body recycles some of its own iron, it still needs to take in an amount from external sources. It is advised that vitamin C be taken at the same time that we eat iron-rich foods. Iron deficiency is common among women, who need 2 mg a day to the 1 mg required by men. It is often indicated for children whose growth rate seems abnormally slow as well as for pregnant women starting in the second trimester of their pregnancy.

Hemochromatosis is the name of the condition caused by an overdose of iron. In instances of hemochromatosis, zinc is prescribed.

A common combination is iron-manganese-copper-cobalt.

Specific properties:

- Acts in the formation of red blood cells, hemoglobin, and myoglobin (the hemoglobin found in our muscles, to which iron brings the oxygen necessary for the muscles to contract)
- Ensures cellular oxygenation
- Plays a role in the synthesis of numerous enzymes (such as peryoxydase and cytochrome)

- Acts as a constituent of catalase, an enzyme that catalyzes the decomposition of oxygenated water in the blood and tissues
- Regularizes growth rate
- Supports the body's immune system
- Counterbalances an excess of phosphorus

Indicated for use in the treatment of:
- Iron-loss anemia from hemorrhage, pregnancy, puberty, menstruation, or convalescence (symptoms of which include fatigue, pallor—especially of the conjunctiva of the eye, lack of wind, palpitations, and dizziness)
- Loss of energy
- Depression
- Menorrhagia
- Sterility
- Hair loss
- Fragile bones
- Soft nails that chip or break easily
- Celiac disease
- Crohn's disease
- AIDS

Lanthanum (La)

Lanthanum is a rare earth. Although its specific properties have yet to be determined (a difficult task in the case of rare earths that are present in our body's tissues in such miniscule amounts), studies have shown that its consumption in very small amounts (lower even than those of trace elements) doubled the life expectancy of lab animals. Some researchers have found lanthanum to be effective in treating intraocular hypertension.

Lead (Pb)

Indicated for cancer
Lead transforms the body's internal cellular environment and has no toxic effects when taken in hyper-trace amounts. It is advised that lead be combined with tin-bismuth.

Specific properties:
- Restores the body's cellular environment when it is in a precancerous state
- Acts as an enzymatic inhibitor

Indicated for use in the treatment of:
- Neoplasia
- Syphilis

Lithium (Li)

Indicated for depression

Lithium acts primarily in the brain, where it affects mood, anxiety, nervousness, and sleep problems. A lithium deficiency gradually manifests as insomnia, anguish, stress, and depression. Our daily needs are roughly 1/100 mg. It is not metabolized by the body. The line separating a healthy dose and a toxic dose is quite fine. It is mainly prescribed at the pharmaceutical level for manic depressive psychosis. In the majority of cases it is safest to take lithium as a trace element, in colloidal form, if possible, to avoid any danger of a toxic reaction. Common combinations are lithium-aluminum and lithium-copper-gold-silver.

Specific properties:
- Acts to improve cerebral circulation in the elderly
- Acts as a diuretic in instances of obesity and high blood pressure

Indicated for use in the treatment of:
- Emotional and mental problems: nervosity, anxiety, nervous depression, irritability, moodiness, agitation, aggressiveness, hyperemotionality
- Muscular tension and twitching
- Minor psychological or psychosomatic displays in children and adults
- Minor sleeping problems
- Troubles caused by menopause
- Circulatory problems

Magnesium (Mg)

Indicated for spasms

Magnesium plays a role in a great number of our body's physiological reactions. It comes into play in the metabolizing of lipids, proteins, and glucids and plays a role in blood clotting and cellular permeability. An essential trace element for the activity and balance of our nervous system, it also exercises a significant effect on muscular activity by making it possible for muscles to relax after contracting.

The recommended daily allowance (from food and other sources) is, on average, 5 to 6 mg per kg of body weight. Sometimes, however, a larger dose is necessary: 10 mg for pregnant women; 15 mg per kg of body weight for growing children. A magnesium deficiency is revealed in a number of conditions, including neuromuscular disorders such as spasmophilia, a state of abnormal excitability, and insomnia.

An excessive intake of certain forms of magnesium could adversely affect the kidneys, which is not an issue if the element is taken in colloidal form. All would agree that magnesium is so key to our processes that a deficiency would effectively block our entire system.

Beneficial combinations include magnesium-cobalt and magnesium-copper-gold-silver.

Specific properties:

- Acts as the essential cation indispensable to all forms of life
- Plays a role in the synthesis of hundreds of enzymes
- Acts in some way in most of our physiological functions (respiratory, endocrine, digestive, hepatic, cardiovascular, and so forth)
- Plays a role in metabolizing glucids, lipids, and proteins
- Plays a role in the assimilation of calcium, phosphorus, and potassium, (especially in bones and teeth)
- Acts to prevent secondary calcifications
- Acts as a thermal regulator
- Acts to protect all vitamins, particularly C and E
- Acts as a sedative to relax the nervous system and improve mental equilibrium and sleep quality
- Supports the body's immune system through the stimulation of phagocytosis (the production of antibodies)
- Plays a role in the regulation of cardiac rhythm and muscular contraction
- Counteracts the effects of aging
- Plays a role in the prevention of cancer (especially when taken in colloidal form or as halogenated salts of magnesium)
- Plays a role in maintaining our system's balanced pH

Indicated for use in the treatment of:

- Decalcification
- Demineralization
- Growth disorders
- Osteoporosis
- Pregnancy (lowers or eliminates the risk of premature birth; calms contractions during pregnancy)
- Warts
- Allergies
- Celiac disease
- Hypoglycemia
- Hyperactivity in children
- Spasmophilia, tetany, shiverings, tinglings
- High blood pressure
- Mitral valve prolapse
- Fatigue
- Impotence
- Psychasthenia (obsessive-compulsive disorder)
- Headaches
- Depression
- Dizziness
- Muscular weakness
- Premenstrual syndrome (PMS)
- Endocrine disorders
- Predisposition to arteriosclerosis
- Aging of the skin
- Fragility of the nails and hair
- Problems connected to membranous permeability
- Certain kinds of obesity, water retention, edema
- Digestive and intestinal disorders, constipation, colitis
- Kidney stones (in combination with vitamin B6)
- Glaucoma
- Raynaud's Disease
- Chronic fatigue syndrome

Manganese (Mn)

Indicated for allergies and cancer

Manganese intervenes in numerous enzymatic reactions, particularly in the synthesis of collagen, the metabolism of glucids, and the construction of bone. It is also a transformational agent of the body's intestinal cellular environment with regard to allergic manifestations such as hay fever. Our bodies contain 10 mg. of manganese, mainly in the liver and kidneys. The recommended daily allowance (from diet and other sources) is approximately 8 mg. Soy milk offers a substantial amount of manganese.

Beneficial combinations include manganese-copper, manganese-cobalt, and manganese-B vitamins (vitamin B complex).

Specific properties:
- Acts as a universal antiallergen
- Acts as a catalyst for cellular oxidation
- Plays a role in the synthesis and activation of numerous enzymes
- Plays a role in metabolizing fats and proteins
- Plays a part in determining the amount of iron that is absorbed and assimilated by the body
- Maintains the health of the skin, bones, and cartilage
- Plays an essential role in reproduction (regulates the endocrine glands, lactation, and the production of sexual hormones)
- Supports the body's immune system
- Plays a role in the activation of SOD, an important antioxidant enzyme
- Acts to combat the multiplication of cancerous cells
- Potentializes the actions of vitamins B_1 and E
- Plays a role in the construction of several enzymatic systems
- Activates arginase and alkaline phosphatase

Indicated for use in treating:
- Morning asthenia with a need for activity and fatigue at bedtime
- All arthritic afflictions
- Eczema and other skin irritations and rashes
- Quincke's edema
- Asthma and hay fever
- Spasmodic rhinitis
- Food allergies
- Migraines and neuralgia
- Glycemia, pancreatic disorders
- Conditions of the nervous system, such as irritability and tachycardia

- Hyperchholesterolemia
- Dysmenorrhea
- Hyperthyroidism
- Growth disorders
- Problems associated with puberty
- Problems associated with menopause
- Impotence
- Obesity
- Vision and hearing problems
- Hypertension
- Anemia

Mercury (Hg)
Indicated for urinary infections
Warning: Mercury is toxic. As a trace element, in the form of salts or a hyper-trace element, however, it is a useful agent in the treatment of certain diseases. An effective combination is mercury-arsenic-bismuth.

Specific properties:
- Acts as a cutaneous antiseptic

Indicated for use in the treatment of:
- Genito-urinary infections

Molybdenum (Mo)
Indicated for regulation of nervous equilibrium
According to the World Health Organization, the recommended daily allowance of molybdenum is 200 to 500 mcg. The symptoms of a molybdenum deficiency are linked to a sulfite poisoning.

Specific properties:
- Plays an essential role in the synthesis of proteins
- Plays an essential role in metabolizing iron
- Plays an essential role in metabolizing nitrogen
- Acts in the transformation of purines into uric acid
- Acts to harmonize cellular function
- Acts to reduce the risk of certain asthma attacks
- Acts as a component of several enzymes, such as xanthine oxydase (a metabolic enzyme), and cysteine

- Maintains a healthy nervous system
- Plays an essential role in maintaining healthy buccal flora

Indicated for use in the treatment of:
- Gingivitis, mouth ulcers
- Impotence (especially among elderly men)
- Cancer

Neodymium (Nd)

Neodymium is a rare earth. Although its role in humans has not yet been examined, studies suggest that it doubles the life expectancy of lab animals.

Nickel (Ni)

Indicated for obesity

A transformative agent of the body's internal cellular environment with important biological properties, nickel plays a primary role in catalysis. It is most often used to treat various conditions associated with dyspepsia. Effective combinations include nickel-cobalt and nickel-zinc-cobalt.

Specific properties:
- Acts as a primary agent of catalysis
- Activates the phosphatases of the spleen, and salivary and pancreatic amylases
- Stimulates the salivary glands
- Strengthens and prolongs the hypoglycemiant action of insulin
- Encourages the production of vitamins A and C
- Encourages growth

Indicated for use in the treatment of:
- Diabetes, liver, pancreas, and spleen ailments
- Dyspepsia, bloating, digestive heaviness, somnolence after meals
- Obesity
- Neoplasia (abnormal cell growth that may be precancerous)
- Overexertion
- Colibacillosis (in combination with cobalt)

Osmium (Os)

Indicated for nervous disorders

There is little information concerning this trace element. Some suggest that osmium is necessary to maintaining balance in the nervous system.

Specific properties:
- Maintains balance in the sympathetic nervous system

Indicated for use in the treatment of:
- Stress, nervousness
- Neurovegetative dystonia (panic attacks)

Phosphorus (P)

Indicated for spasmophilia, tetany

Phosphorus is present in the body in the form of phosphates and is principally found in the bones and the blood, though its action is particularly notable on the nervous system. It plays a role in energetic exchanges with the cells. A phosphorus deficiency is generally indicated by a loss of mineral content in the bones, neurological and cardiac problems, excessive nervousness, and permanent stress. An excessive intake of phosphorus can create an imbalance of blood calcium. The ideal calcium-phosphorus ratio should be 2.5-to-1. Taking a colloidal form of phosphorus ensures this balance is maintained. An overall balance among phosphorus, calcium, and magnesium is essential for good health. Our diet—especially dairy products and fortified processed foods—supplies a substantial quantity of the phosphorus we need.

Specific properties:
- Acts as an antispasmodic
- Plays a role in regulating kidney function (as a diuretic)
- Acts as a constituent of the myelin that covers the nerves
- Ensures effective use of vitamins
- Acts to help the body transform food into energy

Indicated for use in the treatment of:
- Problems in metabolizing calcium
- Growth problems
- In children, problems with the growth of new teeth
- Dystrophy of the bone
- Osteoporosis
- Parathyroid disorders
- Spasmophilia, tetany, cramps and spasms
- Neurovegetative dystonia
- Asthma and respiratory spasms

- Myasthenia
- Dupuytren's Disease
- Scleroderma (an autoimmune disease of the connective tissue)
- Problems with cell growth
- Irregular cardiac rhythm, primarily asystolia (cardiac arrest)
- Cerebral asthenia
- **Contraindicated** for those suffering from acute tuberculosis

Platinum (Pt)

Indicated for cancer treatments

This trace element breaks down oxygenated fluid and opposes its formation on the cellular level where the body has been exposed to x-rays. A powerful catalyst in both the chemical and biological sense, it is a valuable adjunct to treating cancers and those who are genetically predisposed to develop cancer.

Specific properties:

- Acts as an adjunct to cancer treatments, especially radiation therapy, by reducing the harmful effects of these treatments on the body's tissues

Indicated for use in the treatment of:

- Diabetes

Potassium (K)

Indicated for muscle cramps, overexertion

Potassium is present throughout the entire body, particularly the muscle cells, and is integrally involved in the body's fluid balance. It also intervenes in the mechanisms controlling muscle contraction. A potassium deficiency, or hypokalemia, is manifested primarily by muscle cramps, cardiac arythmia, water retention, and high blood pressure. This deficiency is particularly common in cases of intellectual or athletic overexertion, alcoholism, a diet that is too high in coffee and refined sugar, or with the use of diuretics or laxatives or the prolonged use of corticosteroids. Our daily requirement is roughly 400 to 600 mg, but today's foods tend to provide an excess of this element. (Commercial fruits and vegetables are practically force-fed potassium-based fertilizers!) Taking potassium when it is not indicated or required is not only dangerous, it can be fatal. Unless it is taken in as a trace element within a balanced, naturally occurring colloidal form, it should be taken only under the supervision of a trained medical professional.

It should be noted that tobacco and caffeine hinder the assimilation of potassium.

To facilitate diuresis, the advised combination is iodine-potassium-lithium-phosphorus.

Specific properties:
- Regulates cardiac rhythm and blood pressure
- Regulates the suprarenal function
- Regularizes neuromuscular function
- Aids in metabolizing water (works in concert with sodium to control the balance of bodily fluids)
- Acts as a diuretic
- Maintains general mineral balance at a stable weight
- Acts to firm skin and improves its texture
- Acts to improve cerebral oxygenation
- Acts to protect the nervous system

Indicated for use in the treatment of:
- Overexertion
- Muscle fatigue
- Water retention, edema, obesity caused by water retention
- Muscle and skin afflictions
- Rheumatism, arthritis, chronic developing rheumatism, chronic developing polyarthritis, myasthenia
- Chronic diarrhea, prolonged vomiting, and loss of bodily fluids

Praseodymium (Pr)

Praseodymium is a rare earth. Studies have shown that this, like other rare earths, seems to double the life expectancy of laboratory animals.

Radium (Ra)

Our bodies contain a very small amount of this substance. Nothing is yet known about the role of this substance.

Rubidium (Rb)

Indicated for neuromuscular problems

Some believe that this element might play a very import role in transmembranous and cellular transportation, particularly on the level of the central nervous system at the neuromuscular motor end plates. Blood contains a notable amount of rubidium (3.15 mg per liter).

Indicated for use in the treatment of:
- End-plate sclerosis
- Muscle pain
- Myasthenia
- Multiple sclerosis
- Tetany, spasmophilia

Samarium (Sm)

Samarium is another rare earth and, like its counterparts, has been shown to double the normal life expectancy of laboratory animals.

Indicated for use in the treatment of:
- Pylorus problems
- Gastric disorders
- Hiatal hernia

Selenium (Se)

Indicated for premature aging

A metalloid closely related to sulfur, selenium's quantities in the body equal from 3 to 20 mg, which is mainly located in the muscles, bones, and liver. Its action is essentially concentrated on protecting cells from the attack of free radicals, a source of premature aging. This is a particularly relevant indication in today's world, where stress, pollution, and excessive exposure to the sun exact a price.

Its importance, particularly as an anti-aging trace element, is increasingly recognized. Researchers believe that a deficiency of selenium encourages the appearance of more virulent viruses. In fact, recent research (published in 2001) indicates that a selenium deficiency facilitates the appearance of other viruses in animals who have already been infected by viral flu.

This element is not synthesized by the body; thus we depend entirely on diet (which is itself increasingly depleted) for the supply we need. The recommended daily allowance ranges from 60 to 75 mcg, or 1 mcg per kg of body weight, though amounts may reach as high as

200 mcg in instances of the presence of a cancerous or precancerous condition. It is toxic in amounts higher than 500 mcg a day. A selenium deficiency generally announces itself in the premature aging of the body's tissues (particularly that of the skin and heart), difficulties with motor skills, a tendency toward cataracts and cancer, and memory loss. A serious deficiency results in a cardiomyopathy known as Keshan's Disease.

Effective combinations in the case of neoplasy include selenium-copper, selenium-copper-gold-silver, and selenium-uranium-platinum.

Specific properties:
- Prompts important transformations in general metabolism
- Stimulates all exchanges
- Increases diuresis and the elimination of uric acid
- Inhibits the oxygenation of lipids
- Protects fertility
- Boosts thyroid function in the event of hyperthyroidism
- Plays a role in eliminating heavy toxic metals (cadmium, lead, aluminum, mercury) from the body (as an antioxidant)
- Plays a role in eliminating free radicals from the body
- Plays a role in removing age spots from the skin
- Plays a role in the construction of glutathion-peroxydase (an antioxidant enzyme that helps in the fight against oxidative stress and protects against cancer)
- Acts to prevent cardiovascular disease and heart attack
- Acts to prevent myopathy (muscle disorders)
- Destroys cancerous tissue
- Combats chemotherapy's side effects
- Supports the body's immune system
- Protects from cancer
- Supports the function of the suprarenal glands
- Protects the liver from the risk of cirrhosis
- Protects the pancreas

Indicated for use in the treatment of:
- Mycosis, acne (preferably combined with sulfur)
- AIDS
- Cancer
- Cancerous tissue

- Macular degeneration, retinopathy, cataracts
- Prostate problems (especially when combined with vitamin E and zinc)

Silicon (Si)
Indicated for premature aging
Organic silicon—such as that found in horsetail, which has been rendered naturally bioavailable by other elements in the plant that combine with it—should never be confused with man-made silicon, which, in the form of asbestos (hydrated silicate of calcium and magnesium), for instance, is highly toxic. In its colloidal form silicon has a wide array of beneficial properties that affect the entire body. The regenerative properties of organic silicon on the cell are well-known, thanks to the successful research of French professor Norbert Duffaut.

Silicon acts as antidote to aluminum, which is toxic when not in colloidal form. Effective combinations include silicon-boron, silicon-calcium, silicon-magnesium, silicon-manganese, and silicon-potassium.

Specific properties:
- Regenerates bone, skin, nails, and hair
- Plays a role in demineralization and decalcification
- Encourages the formation of bone collagen and connective tissue
- Encourages assimilation of calcium in the early stages of bone growth
- Acts to balance the nervous system
- Encourages the formation of the endocrine glands
- Rehydrates skin and mucous membranes
- Promotes healing of tissue
- Acts to strengthen the walls of the arteries and helps them retain their flexibility
- Prevents cardiovascular disease
- Prevents Alzheimer's disease
- Prevents osteoporosis
- Supports the body's immune system

Indicated for use in the treatment of:
- Osteoporosis
- Slow growth

- Premature aging
- Arteriosclerosis
- Stretch marks
- Cerebral atonia, loss of concentration and memory
- Osteritis, adenopathy (swollen lymph nodes)
- Prostate problems
- Hypertension
- High cholesterol
- Warts

Silver (Ag)

Indicated for bacterial and viral infection

Silver is an agent of change in the internal cellular environment that is especially active against viral infections occurring in the ORL sphere. It has long been known for its antiseptic properties. Indeed, our grandparents knew that soaking a silver ring or other silver object in water would transform the liquid into an excellent preservative.

It is commonly combined with other trace elements (silver-copper, silver-gold).

Specific properties:
- Acts as a powerful antiviral agent and bactericide
- Acts to reduce fever

Indicated for use in the treatment of:
- Puerperal infections (those following childbirth)
- Metritis
- Cystitis with colon bacillis or gonococcus
- Staphylococcia (especially in combination with tin)
- Septicemia
- Pneumonia (especially in combination with selenium)
- Grippe (especially in combination with copper)
- Angina (especially in combination with bismuth)
- Acute joint rheumatism
- Buccal ulcers
- Inflammation
- Cancer (silver salts seem to have an analgesic effect on cancer pain)
- Combinations: copper-gold-silver, manganese-copper

Sodium (Na)

Indicated for regulation of bodily fluids

The elderly and the very young are the most vulnerable to a lack of salt because their thirst mechanism is either not regulated (in the former) or is still immature (in the latter). Thus these two groups run a greater risk of dehydration when temperatures are high. As for the rest of us, it is clear that most of us consume far too much sodium, so only in exceptional instances is it useful to increase our consumption. Sodium in a colloidal form, however, can support certain regulating processes. It is necessary for our bodies to maintain a proper balance of potassium and sodium—an excess of one causes a deficiency in the other, which can eventually lead to heart problems.

Specific properties:
- Plays an essential role in metabolizing water
- Balances blood pH and the body's acid-alkaline balance
- Encourages digestion and elimination
- Plays an essential role in healthy nerve and muscle function
- Regularizes the quantity of bodily fluids (blood, for instance, contains roughly 10 g of sodium per liter)
- Acts to regulate heart rhythm

Strontium (Sr)

Indicated for osteoporosis

Only infinitesimal traces of this can be found in the body.

Specific properties:
- Supports bone resistance
- Prevents tooth decay

Indicated for use in the treatment of:
- Bone lesions, especially those of cancerous origin (reduces pain)

Sulfur (S)

Indicated for promoting healthy skin and joints

Widely present throughout the body, the trace element sulfur, among other things, acts on the skin, hair, nails, and cartilage. It ensures that the joints maintain their flexibility and helps reduce joint pain. In addition, sulfur regulates the internal cellular environment by helping in the fight against winter ailments.

Specific properties:
- Potentializes the actions of all other elements (according to Dr. Picard)
- Plays an essential role in the construction of numerous proteins, including those responsible for hair, muscle, and skin growth
- Regulates hepato-biliary function
- Acts as a general anti-allergen
- Acts as a basic building block of amino acids such as methionine, cysteine, taurine, thiamin, and glutathione, heparin, keratin, and chondroitin sulfate acid
- Acts as a constituent of bones, teeth, and collagen
- Acts as a blood purifier
- Protects against toxic substances that may be present on the blood (such as heavy metals)
- Protects against the harmful effects of radiation and pollution
- Acts as an anti-aging agent
- Acts as a constituent of insulin; encourages the regulation of glycemia

Indicated for use in the treatment of:
- Eczema, skin rashes, recurring skin disorders, dermatosis, acne
- Hay fever, allergic asthma
- Infection
- Arthritis, rheumatism, osteoarthritis
- Asthma
- Migraines
- Hepatic insufficiency
- Recurring ailments of the ORL sphere

Tellurium (Te)

We know that tellurium is found in the body but know nothing of its properties, though some suggest that it acts to promote cerebral circulation, prevents hepatic disorders, and prevents nightmares.

Thulium (Tm)

Thulium is a rare earth. Like all other rare earths, it seems to double the normal life expectancy of lab animals.

Tin (Tn)

Indicated for infections and staphylococci

Colloidal tin, in contrast to salts, has no toxicity. It is effective against all infections and staphylococci. One sign of a deficiency in this element is male baldness.

Specific properties:
- Acts as an anti-infectant
- Supports the body's immune system
- Encourages new hair growth
- Prevents deafness
- Improves reflexes
- Plays a role in numerous bio-electrical functions (especially in combination with lead-bismuth)

Indicated for use in the treatment of:
- Staphylococci (especially in combination with copper)
- Abscesses, boils, acne
- Anthrax
- Cancer
- Syphilis

Titanium (Ti)

The human body contains an average of 0.1 to 2 mg per kg of titanium. We do not yet know much about its physiological effects.

Uranium (U)

Indicated for shortcircuiting cellular proliferation

Uranium alters the internal cellular environment directly at the cellular level. It also stimulates the immune system defenses and improves digestion. It completes the defiltering action of copper by acting against cellular proliferation related to tumors or cancer. An effective combination for fighting cancer is uranium-gold.

Specific properties
- Acts against cellular proliferations
- Revitalizes tissue and accelerates healing

Indicated for use in the treatment of:
- Cancer (as salts)
- Skin exposed to radiation therapy
- Dyspepsia

Vanadium (V)

Indicated for bone and tooth growth

The daily requirement for vanadium is roughly 100 mcg. It is present in small amounts in products of animal origin. A recent study on insulin-dependent diabetes undertaken at the Vancouver Medical School in British Columbia showed evidence that at certain dosages this trace element replaced insulin and encouraged the regeneration of pancreatic tissue that had been damaged by chromium and vanadium deficiencies.

Chromium and vanadium are antagonists, thus they must be taken at different times of the day—unless they are taken in the form of a colloidal water complex, in which they are naturally balanced.

Specific properties:
- Contributes to the fixing of calcium in the bones
- Plays a role in cellular metabolism
- Plays an essential role in the formation of bones and teeth
- Prevents tooth decay
- Encourages growth
- Aids in reproduction and fertility
- Plays an important role in the metabolism of lipids (inhibits the synthesis of cholesterol
- Protects against cancer and cardio-vascular diseases

Indicated for use in the treatment of:
- Non-insulin-dependent diabetes
- Difficulty with kidney function
- Impotence, sterility
- Neoplasia

Ytterbium (Yb)

Ytterbium is another rare earth about which little is known.

Yttrium (Y)

Yttrium is also a rare earth and, like the others, seems to double the normal life expectancy of laboratory animals. Some health specialists have recommended this element for use in the treatment of eye disorders and vision problems and a weakened immune system.

Zinc (Zn)

Indicated for trouble with ovarian function and the prostate

Zinc was well-known in ancient times, when it was used in the treatment of burns and wounds. It is also a natural antioxidant with a wealth of benefits. Zinc is involved in numerous enzymatic reactions (more than 200!), especially those playing a role in the synthesis of proteins. It is especially active on the level of the phaneres (nails and hair) and the skin. It also plays a role in the production of hair keratin and collagen. Zinc also strongly boosts the immune system. Other noteworthy effects include a positive effect on growth, the regulation of insulin, and sexual hormonal mechanisms. It is also known for its role in determining the integrity of genetic paternity (what is known in molecular biology as "zinc fingers," a sequence of twenty amino acids arranged in a way that resembles the fingers of a glove. These are connected to a zinc atom that gives protein the ability to interact with DNA).

The human body contains about 2 grams of zinc. The recommended daily allowance (from food and other sources) about 5 to 10 mg for children, 30 to 50 mg for pregnant women and nursing mothers, and 25 to 30 mg for the average adult. In its colloidal form it plays an essential role in balancing all elements. It is important to make sure that young children, pregnant women, and the elderly are not suffering from a zinc deficiency. Its absorption is hindered by excess calcium and it competes with copper. This risk is eliminated when it is taken in its trace element, colloidal form. There are multiple consequences for a zinc deficiency, which include: changes in the skin (greasy skin, inflammation, eczema, dermitis), loss of hair, wounds do not readily heal, growth problems (in children), weakened immune system, susceptibility to infections, sexual problems, and problems with the sense of taste.

Zinc deficiency often causes the appearance of white spots on the nails.

Deficiency can be due to a number of different factors such as smoking, alcoholism, drinking too much coffee, taking diuretics, and eating a diet that is too rich in refined foods. The first symptom of a deficiency is generally a loss of the senses of smell and taste.

Effective combinations include zinc-copper, for endocrine problems occurring during puberty and slow growth, and zinc-nickel-cobalt, as a hypoglycemiant.

Specific properties:

- Plays an essential role in the mature growth of the sexual organs such as the ovaries and testicles, and in the synthesis of sex hormones (testosterone and prostaglandins)
- Regulates the hypophysial functions (those related to the pituitary gland)
- Prevents the risk of congenital abnormalities
- Promotes healing of wounds
- Stimulates the production of T lymphocytes (white blood cells)
- Plays an essential role in the growth and coloration of hair
- Strengthens bones
- Supports hepatic function and protects the liver from toxins
- Prevents acne
- Regulates activity of the sebaceous glands
- Plays an essential role in the synthesis of keratin and collagen
- Plays a role in the synthesis of proteins (activates RNA polymerases) and the assimilation of proteins and glucids in the digestive tract
- Plays a role in the storing and availability of glucose in the cells
- Acts to neutralize excess copper
- Governs the acid-alkaline balance of the body
- Maintains balance in the sympathetic nervous system
- Acts as a constituent (as coenzyme) of more than 300 enzymes (including SOD— superoxide dismutase—which plays a crucial role in the fight against aging, as well as carbonic anhydrase, alcohol dehydrogenase, and the carboxypeptidases of the pancreas)
- Supports the body's immune system
- Plays a role in the synthesis of DNA

- Encourages olfactory and gustatory acuteness
- Acts as a powerful antioxidant
- Plays an essential role in the activity of certain vitamins (makes it possible for the proper concentration of vitamin E to be maintained in the blood; improves assimilation of vitamin A

Indicated for use in the treatment of:
- At-risk pregnancies
- Depression
- Alopecia, hair loss, premature graying of hair
- Acne
- Crohn's disease
- Peptic ulcers
- Chronic lesions in the teguments (20 percent of zinc is found in the teguments—natural protective coverings of the body; lesions here are a result of its deficiency)
- Fatigue, hair loss, impotence
- Poor night vision
- White spots on the nails
- Defective memory

Appendix I

EXCERPTS FROM U.S. SENATE DOCUMENT 264, 74TH CONGRESS, SECOND SESSION, 1936

Do you know that most of us today are suffering from certain dangerous diet deficiencies, which cannot be remedied until the depleted soils from which our foods come are brought into proper mineral balance?

The alarming fact is that foods—fruits and vegetables and grains—now being raised on millions of acres of land that no longer contain enough of certain needed minerals, are starving us, no matter how much of them we eat!

You'd think, wouldn't you, that a carrot is a carrot—that one is about as good as another as far as nourishment is concerned. But it isn't; one carrot may look and taste like another and yet be lacking in the particular mineral element which our system requires and which carrots are supposed to contain. Laboratory tests prove that the fruits, the vegetables, the grains, the eggs, and even the milk and the meats of today are not what they were a few generations ago. (Which doubtless explains why our forefathers thrived on a selection of foods that would starve us!) No man of today can eat enough fruits and vegetables to supply his system with the mineral salts he requires for perfect health, because his stomach isn't big enough to hold them! And we are running to big stomachs.

No longer does a balanced and fully nourishing diet consist merely of so many calories of certain vitamins or a fixed proportion of starches, proteins, and carbohydrates. We now know that it must contain, in addition, something like a score of mineral salts.

It is bad news to learn from our leading authorities that 99 percent of the American people are deficient in these minerals, and that a marked deficiency in anyone of the more important minerals actually results in disease. Any upset of the balance, any considerable lack of one or another element, however microscopic the body requirement may be, and we sicken, suffer, shorten our lives.

This discovery is one of the latest and most important contributions of science to the problem of human health.

"Bear in mind," says Dr. Northen, "that minerals are vital to human metabolism and health—and that no plant or animal can appropriate to itself any mineral which is not present in the soil upon which it feeds.

"We know that vitamins are complex chemical substances which are indispensable to nutrition, and that each of them is of importance for the normal function of some special structure in the body. Disorder and disease result from any vitamin deficiency.

"It is not commonly realized, however, that vitamins control the body's appropriation of minerals, and in the absence of minerals they have no function to perform. Lacking vitamins, the system can make some use of minerals, but lacking minerals, vitamins are useless.

"The truth is that our foods vary enormously in value, and some of them aren't worth eating, as food.

"Some of our lands, even in a virgin state, never were well-balanced in mineral content, and unhappily for us, we have been systematically robbing the poor soils and the good soils alike of the very substances most necessary to health, growth, long life, and resistance to disease."

We know that rats, guinea pigs, and other animals can be fed into a diseased condition and out again by controlling only the minerals in their food.

A 10-year test with rats proved that by withholding calcium they can be bred down to a third the size of those fed with an adequate amount of that mineral. Their intelligence, too, can be controlled by mineral feeding as readily as can their size, their bony structure, and their general health.

Place a number of these little animals inside a maze after starving some of them of a certain mineral element. The starved ones will be unable to find their way out, whereas the others will have little or no difficulty in getting out. Their dispositions can be altered by mineral feeding. They can be made quarrelsome and belligerent; they can even be turned into cannibals and be made to devour each other.

A cage of normal rats will live in amity. Restrict their calcium, and they will become irritable and draw apart from one another. Then they will begin to fight. Restore their calcium balance and they will grow friendlier; in time they will begin to sleep in a pile as before.

Many backward children are "stupid" merely because they are deficient in magnesia [magnesium]. We punish them for our failure to feed them properly.

Certainly our physical well-being is more directly dependent upon the mineral we take into our systems than upon calories or vitamins or upon the precise proportions of starch, protein, or carbohydrates we consume.

It is now agreed that at least 16 mineral elements are indispensable for normal nutrition, and several more are always found in small amounts in the body, although their precise physiological role has not been determined. Of the 11 indispensable salts, calcium, phosphorus, and iron are perhaps the most important.

Here's one specific example: The soil around a certain midwest city is poor in calcium. Three hundred children of this community were examined and nearly 90 percent had bad teeth. Sixty-nine percent showed affections of the nose and throat, swollen glands, enlarged or diseased tonsils. More than one-third had defective vision, round shoulders, bow legs, and anemia.

So it goes, down through the list, each mineral element playing a definite role in nutrition. A characteristic set of symptoms, just as specific as any vitamin-deficiency disease, follows a deficiency in any one of them. It is alarming, therefore, to face the fact that we are starving for these precious, health-giving substances.

The minerals in fruits and vegetables are colloidal; i.e., they are in a state of such extremely fine suspension that they can be assimilated by the human system.

Sick soils mean sick plants, sick animals, and sick people. Physical, mental, and moral fitness depend largely upon an ample supply and a proper proportion of the minerals in our foods. Nerve function, nerve stability, nerve cell-building likewise depends thereon.

[Dr. Northen states] "Soils seriously deficient in minerals cannot produce plant life competent to maintain our needs, and with the continuous cropping and shipping away of those concentrates, the condition becomes worse.

"A famous nutrition authority recently said, 'One sure way to end the American people's susceptibility to infection is to supply through food a balance ration of iron, copper, and other metals. An organism supplied with a diet adequate to, or preferable in excess of, all mineral requirements may so utilize these elements as to produce immunity from infection quite beyond anything we are able to produce artificially by our present method of immunization. You can't make up the deficiency by using patent medicine.'"

HIMALAYAN CRYSTAL SALT

Himalayan crystal salt was formed 250 millions years ago when the Himalaya Mountains rose up out of the primitive ocean that covered nearly the entire surface of the planet. It is the mineral memory of that original sea.

The salt can be found specifically in a low-lying 200-square mile area in northwest Pakistan situated in the first foothills of the Himalayas. Due to changes in climatic conditions and powerful tectonic movements long ago, the sea covering this region evaporated and the great Himalaya range emerged, which accounts for the existence of these cubic crystalline structures at such high altitudes.

Similar deposits of salt exist in many places in the world, but this Himalayan salt is the only one both formed in such circumstances and sheltered from any traces of atmospheric pollution. It is extracted manually from the earth and is packed on site without any treatment whatsoever.

Himalayan crystal salt is the most beneficial, cleanest salt available on this planet. It is absolutely pristine and natural, identical to the ancient primal ocean from which it originally came. We owe to Professor Peter Ferreira, a German biophysicist who carried out research on colloidal elements and cellular nutrition, the rediscovery of the range its benefits, which prompted him to perform clinical tests on patients who were consuming on a daily basis a salt water solution prepared using Himalayan salt. Some of the results of these studies indicated that patients experienced the disappearance of heavy metals from the body, dissolution of existing calcium deposits, slow and in-depth general detoxification, and the rebalancing of blood pH—exactly the effects of Quinton's Marine Plasma.

Ferreira and his coauthor, Dr. Barbara Hendel, published the results,[1] which subsequently became well-known and were translated into English. The extraordinary interest in Himalayan salt following this publication inevitably brought conflicts between the owners of the mines and those exploring varying theories about the origin of the salt deposits.

Historically, however, Himalayan crystal salt has been known and used for centuries in both Ayurvedic and Tibetan medicine. In addition, for quite some time doctors have employed the energy of this salt, which exists in the form of vital mineral elements locked within its perfectly formed, mineral-rich crystals, to treat with great success almost every disorder known to humans.

Because of its ionized colloidal structure, all of the salt's minerals and trace elements are completely absorbed by the body. When compared to ordinary sea salt under a microscope, we can see that its elements are perfectly linked to the crystal itself, whereas in ordinary sea salt they are dispersed without any links to the crystal.

Just like Quinton's Marine Plasma and T. J. Clark's water from Utah, it contains all the elements found in our bodies—as determined by analysis, at least 84 "natural" elements needed by the body, nearly all 96 trace elements, excluding in part helium, argon, neon, krypton, xenon, and radon, which can be detected only through extremely sophisticated and costly analysis. Today, European doctors and alternative health practitioners alike are successfully applying the ancient knowledge of *sole,* or brine, derived from combining Himalayan crystal salt with good-quality spring water. Their success is worthy of our attention.

But how exactly does Himalayan salt differ from other kinds of salt that we use in our diets? Regular table salt, which is useless as a food and potentially destructive to health, has no vibrant crystalline structure. Instead, it shows only dead crystals that are completely isolated from each other. In order for the body to metabolize these, it must sacrifice tremendous amounts of energy with very little in the way of results. Refined sea salt displays structure but its irregular crystals are isolated and disconnected from the important, vital elements surrounding them. An ionic-colloidal assimilation of the elements thus cannot be guaranteed and many vital minerals the salt may contain cannot be absorbed by the body without its expenditure of a tremendous amount of energy. Net nutritional gains are small with an even greater loss of energy. Natural gray sea salt is much better for us than refined sea salt, though it has not been exempt from exposure to pollution.

Results of research on Himalayan crystal salt only prove how harmoniously it interacts with our makeup and how vital its life-generating power is for our body as a whole and our nervous system particularly. Its balanced crystalline structure reveals fine branching and unlike refined sea salt, the crystal itself is not isolated from its 84+ mineral elements. This tells us that its mineral energy content is balanced and can be easily metabolized by the body. When taken as food, Himalayan crystal salt has a vital, energetic effect on the body. When water is added to it, its stored energy, or biophoton content, is set free. In this crystal salt, with its perfect geometric structure formed geologically over millions of years, the elements are available in such tiny particles and its minerals exist in such an ultimate ionic form that we can easily absorb and metabolize them.

Specifically, Himalayan crystal salt is a powerful antioxidant that works everywhere in the body. The simple reason for this lies in the fact that crystal salt contains in ideal proportions all 72 mineral elements that compose the human body. Due to the immense amount of spare electrons that all of these elements carry in crystal salt, they have great antioxidant properties. Once crystal salt is introduced into the body, a profound regeneration of the cell membranes becomes possible. It also enhances the effectiveness of other antioxidants.

Many European studies have shown that crystal salt contains quantities of calcium and magnesium, two minerals essential for health. Peter Ferreira performed a two-year study on 400 people who used crystal salt and some of his findings indicated that through consumption of the salt, blood pressure could be balanced, calcium deposits could be eliminated, usable oxygen in the blood could be increased, red blood cells could be separated, and blood could be detoxified. In addition, his study indicated that the full spectrum of elements that resonate with our bones and enzymes and that build bone marrow could be utilized; radiation could be neutralized; capillaries could become more elastic, which increases blood flow; and extra electrons, super-antioxidant free- radical scavengers, could be added to the body. But that's not all: The entire range of electrolytes needed by the body could be received, uric acid could be detoxified from sodium chloride intake, heavy metals could possibly be eliminated through the stool, and cravings for sweets could be reduced. In short, this healthful, delicious, beautiful, pink salt added to our diet could also add to our life and health.

Using Himalayan salt is easy. It is simply excellent as a table salt—a wholesome product with no chemical additives that has not been refined in any way. Interestingly, it seems that it does not have the same negative consequences to human health as those frequently attributed to ordinary salt. Naturally, this does not mean that it can be consumed in excess. Only a small amount per day is necessary to provide all the colloidal elements we need for good health.

GENERAL APPLICATIONS

Bathing

The therapeutic use of salt in the bath for its regenerating, purifying, and detoxifying action has a long history and continues to be well-known today. Of all the different types of bath salts available, Himalayan salt seems to have the most powerful effects. It imparts a feeing of well-being and peacefulness together with an intense muscular relaxation. Some have even claimed that use of these salts in baths has reduced their need for antidepressants and sleep-inducing drugs.

Be alert, however, to the surprising effects that their strength of action can produce after a bath, especially for the first few times of use. Agitation, boosted energy, or a state of total exhaustion can occur simultaneously with the disappearance of pain in the joints, soothing of common skin complaints, and occasional dizziness. In the beginning it is best to try a bath with these salts on the evening preceding a day off from work.

It is also important to remember that metabolic reactions to these salts can differ from one person to the next and that even if some effects might seem negative at first, it is perfectly harmless to continue bathing in Himalayan salts. Through such bathing the salts can rebalance the body by bringing to it the elements necessary for the catalytic processes within cellular metabolism and by acting as a vector for energy thanks to its ionic (electric) activity. When the body is immersed in a salt-and-water solution, metabolic processes are stimulated and the body actually assimilates the minerals and colloidal trace elements present in the salt, which can be confirmed by measuring urinary pH before and after bathing. Usually we can discern a correction in the body's acidity. In addition, because the bath provides optimal hydration and purification, the skin is also improved and invigorated.

Application: Place about 1 pound of salt crystals in the bathtub, if your tub is large. (This results in a 1 percent salt concentration—the same as the medium in the body's cells, thus ideal for exchange.) Cover the salt with a little water and allow it to dissolve, then fill the bathtub with water at 98.6°F (body temperature). Soak in this solution for 15 to 20 minutes. After bathing, do not towel dry; allow the skin to air dry. Bathe in this solution a maximum of 2 times per week.

Contraindication: If you have any heart conditions or are pregnant, avoid this type of bath.

Rhythm Bathing

Observations have shown that the best results can be achieved from taking a Himalayan salt bath at specific times during the cycle of the moon. On the day of the full moon, the absorption potential of the body, and therefore the potential for the salt's effectiveness, is at its peak. At this time the body will absorb most of the minerals from the salt bath as they penetrate the skin in the form of ions. The body's bioenergetic weak points are harmonized and its own energy flow is activated.

At the time of the new moon, the body's capacity for detoxification is at its highest. This is a perfect time for a cleansing salt bath. At this time we can easily withstand weight adjustment and decontamination of the body.

Application: Add 2 pounds of salt crystals to the bathtub with enough water to dissolve the crystals, and leave this solution for approximately 1 hour. Then fill the tub with warm water at about 98.6° F. Do not add any other chemicals or products to the bath. Bathe 15 to 20 minutes, then allow your skin to air dry.

Sole (Brine) Drinking Therapy

Usually 1 teaspoon of diluted salt water is adequate for therapeutic effect without provoking a significant increase in daily salt consumption. This kind of treatment supplies the body with essential minerals and trace elements, rebalances pH, improves digestion, assists in the elimination of toxins and deposits, and rids the body of heavy metals.

Application: Loosely fill a closeable glass container with several Himalayan salt crystals. Add spring water or "enlivened" water, completely filling the vessel. If the crystals have dissolved after approximately 24 hours, add a few more. When the water is no longer able to dissolve salt, there will be salt crystals sitting at the bottom of the jar. At this point the solution will be saturated at approximately 26 percent, the appropriate saturation for a sole solution. This concentration is stable and can be kept indefinitely. The container can be refilled again and again with water and salt to the same point of saturation.

Each morning before breakfast, drink 1 teaspoon of the sole water mixed with 250 ml of spring water.

Body Peel

This mixture of pure Himalayan salt and oil applied to the skin is ideal for its detoxifying and energizing effects. You will achieve the same purifying result as from fasting for several days, but at the same time the body will receive an energy boost from the highly concentrated minerals in the salt mixture. The application of this mixture also enhances blood circulation in the skin.

Application: In a small bowl mix until smooth $3^1/2$ tablespoons of pure Himalayan salt crystals, 1 tablespoon of macadamia nut oil, and $^1/4$ teaspoon of 100 percent pure lavender oil. Next, take a warm shower to open the pores, then lie on a bath towel and rub your entire body with the salt mixture. You will experience deeper relaxation if somebody else does this for you. Wrap yourself in the towel then cover yourself with a blanket. Keep the peeling compress on for about 30 minutes. You will slowly feel a warm glow throughout your body, indicating that the body's cells have begun their work. Rinse off the mixture with warm water and gently pat dry the skin.

SPECIFIC THERAPEUTIC INDICATIONS FOR HIMALAYAN SALT

Arthritis and Gout

On an empty stomach drink 1 teaspoon of sole (see Sole Drinking Therapy, above) mixed with spring water. Continue drinking at least 2 to 3 quarts of spring water throughout the day.

A cold poultice made from a pure sole solution (26 percent) can also bring some relief. Apply this to affected areas and wrap each with a dry cloth bandage.

Osteoporosis

On an empty stomach drink 1 teaspoon of sole (see Sole Drinking Therapy, above) mixed with spring water. Continue drinking at least 2 to 3 quarts of water throughout the day.

Additionally, you can make a warm-water sole poultice containing a 10 percent concentration of sole (1/2 ounce to 4 ounces of water) and apply it to sore joints or other sore body parts. Or fill a linen or cotton bag with salt crystals and heat it in the microwave to 125–140°F. Place the heated bag directly on your sore joints or other sore body part for 20 minutes. If joint pains occur in you hands and feet, you can also bathe these extremities in a more concentrated sole solution, starting at 10 percent. A water temperature that mimics body temperature (98.6°F) is ideal for this application.

Asthma and Bronchitis

On an empty stomach, drink 1 teaspoon of sole mixed with spring water. Continue drinking at least 2 to 3 quarts of water throughout the day.

Additional applications: Heat 4 to 8 quarts of water to the boiling point. Add 1 ounce of Himalayan salt for each quart of water and let it dissolve. Cover your head with a towel and inhale the steam for 10 to 15 minutes, keeping your face far enough away from the hot steam to avoid being scalded. Continue this therapy once or twice a day.

Open Wounds

To treat these, use a poultice made of sole: Soak a sterile gauze in a sole solution of ½ ounce of Himalayan salt diluted in ½ cup of high-quality, noncarbonated mineral water (a higher salt-to-water ratio will produce a burning sensation in the injured area). Squeeze the excess water from the gauze, apply it to the wound, and wrap a cloth around it to hold it in place.

Detoxification for Flu and Fever Relief

Mix a 3 percent sole solution of 2 tablespoons Himalayan crystal salt dissolved in 1 quart of water. Soak a shirt thoroughly in this solution, then wring it out, put it on, wrap yourself in a dry towel, and lie in bed, covered with a blanket. After about 30 minutes you will start perspiring profusely. Drink a cup of linden or lime blossom tea and remain in bed for another 60 to 90 minutes. Remove the shirt, rinse yourself in the shower, and treat yourself to 1 hour of rest.

This procedure detoxifies the body and activates metabolism. In cases of flu it produces better results than a sole-solution bath. If you suffer from flu, cold feet, or gout, you may also soak a pair of clean cotton socks in a 3 to 5 percent sole solution mixed from 2 to 4 tablespoons of Himalayan salt diluted in 1 quart of water, wring the socks thoroughly, put them on, then wrap your feet in a dry towel. After about 60 minutes, remove the socks, rinse your feet, and treat yourself to 1 hour of rest.

For inhalation, in a pot heat 2 quarts of water to the boiling point, then add 1 ounce of salt and let it dissolve. Breathe in the steam for 15 to 20 minutes to clear and soothe the upper respiratory tract.

Dental Hygiene

Healthy teeth and gums are not only visually appealing but are also very important to our overall health. Most common tooth problems derive from excess acidity in the mouth and throat. A sole solution of Himalayan salt builds up mouth flora with a neutral pH and helps to protect tooth enamel.

Brush your teeth every morning with the concentrated sole solution, using your tongue to help work the solution through your teeth. After spitting out this solution, gargle with fresh sole for about 3 minutes, then spit it out again.

Psoriasis

Psoriasis is often inherited and mostly appears in adulthood. The disease, however, does not have to last for a lifetime. An alkaline diet including fresh or frozen vegetables (with the exception of Brussels sprouts and artichokes), salads, mushrooms, fresh fruits, potatoes, all other root vegetables, top-grade olive oil, fruit and vegetable juices, water and herbal teas, and abstinence from animal proteins is the foundation for treatment. Salt therapy imparts additional beneficial effects. In fact, for quite a long time traditional medicine has recognized the healing power of salt in the treatment of psoriasis.

Every morning before breakfast, drink a mixture of 1 teaspoon of sole solution and a glass of water, then drink 2 to 3 quarts of spring water throughout the day. Combine this therapy with a 10–20 minute salt bath taken 2 times per week. Begin with a 3 percent sole solution made by diluting about 6 pounds of Himalayan salt crystals in a tub full of water that is no higher than 98.6°F. If possible, allow yourself to dry in the sun. In subsequent baths, gradually increase the concentration to 8 percent. The sole bath acts to moisturize your skin and stop inflammation. The parts of the body that can be more severely affected by psoriasis, such as the elbows and knees, can be massaged directly with a 26 percent sole solution.

Herpes

Herpes sores are very painful, annoying, and persistent. Once you have been infected with the virus, it resides permanently in the nervous system. As soon as the immune system is weakened, it can become activated, multiplying at an explosive rate and forming the well-known blisters. Once they appear, usual remedies offer little relief. The intake of a sole solution strengthens the immune system to help prevent outbreaks.

On an empty stomach, drink 1 teaspoon of sole solution mixed with spring water. Continue drinking at least 2 to 3 quarts of spring water throughout the day. To treat blisters, with a cotton swab apply a 26 percent concentrated sole solution directly to the affected site every hour.

Appendix 3

TRIBOMECHANICALLY ACTIVATED ZEOLITES (TMAZs)

Lycopenomin, a mineral preparation and dietary food supplement that has recently appeared on the market,* is generating interest within the scientific and professional community as a result of its surprisingly positive effects, particularly among those suffering from severe chronic diseases.

The results of scientific studies of the effects of this product, particularly its basic components, *tribomechanically activated zeolites,* or *clinoptilolites*—also called TMAZ—have shown their strong antioxidative effects, their ability to absorb heavy metals and toxins, and their ability to bring into balance an organism that has lost its equilibrium. Since 1997, through scientific research and observations of patients in Croatia, Austria, Germany and the United States, valuable data has been collected on the effects of this mineral product.

Zeolite is a generic term for a family of volcanic rocks whose natural

---

*Lycopenomin Active® is a dietary supplement manufactured by Megamin GmbH, Berlin, Germany and now distributed in the United States (see appendix 4). It is composed of lycopene, vitamin C, selenium and the tribomechanically micronized natural mineral clinoptilolite. Based on known biological properties of its ingredients, Lycopenomin Active® is intended to maintain a proper balance of essential and trace minerals, to stimulate immune response, and to provide antioxidative protection.

environment is volcanic formations and cliffs that have been sedimented both in the ocean and by gas and steam. Zeolites are natural microporous silicate minerals ranging in color from colorless to white or light red, possibly due to the presence of impurities and traces of other minerals. In composition they are Al-Na or Al-Ca silicates and when heated they foam and seem to melt. There are three known types of zeolites: fibrous zeolite, leafy zeolite, and crystalline zeolite, which together occur naturally in 106 variations.

The crystalline zeolite clinoptilolite has been selected for tribomechanical processing in a patented instrument because of its characteristic ease of absorption and selectivity and its ion exchange capacity. This mineral is completely safe for human use and consumption, as has been demonstrated through chemical analyses and toxicological studies.

Specifically, a clinoptilolite from the Kozark area of Slovakia was selected for the production of TMAZ. Microscopically, the mineral is found to contain very fine grains of radial zeolite. It is a typical tuffaceous mineral mainly consisting of volcanic glass, which later has been recrystalized. Recent results have demonstrated that zeolite is a major antioxidant, a glucose adsorbent, and a potential adjuvant in anticancer therapy.[1]

The term TMAZ applies to natural zeolites from the clinoptilolite group processed in a vortical centrifugal micronization machine. As determined by X-ray analysis performed on samples before and after activation, this process does not cause changes in the chemical composition of natural mineral zeolite. The tribomechanical activation procedure does, however, alter the physicochemical properties of natural zeolite to a significant degree. The most significant changes occur in its particle size, active surface, electrostatic charge, and ion exchange capacity. In comparison to nonactivated zeolite, the average TMAZ particle size is about 6 times smaller. TMAZ also has greater ion exchange capacity than nonactivated zeolite.

Tribomechanical activation does not merely vary the size of the particles but also produces a fragmented and irregular surface on each of them and, consequently, a new distribution of electrons on the surface of the mineral. In the tribomechanical activator the mineral particles undergo 3,000 collisions per second at speeds of up to three times the speed of sound. The particles explode against each other, producing granulometric readings toward the nanoparticle—a millionth of a millimeter—and a fragmented, irregular surface with great active potential.

But where did the process that produces TMAZ originate? After thirty years of research on mineral activation, Professor Tihomir Lelas perfected the revolutionary process called tribomechanical activation or TMA, using air-draft propulsion. Through this process mineral particles are reduced to a dimension between a micron and a few nanometers using tens of thousands of high speed collisions with other particles. The result is a mineral powder with a greatly increased active surface. In fact, when the size of the particles is divided by 10, the active surface is multiplied by 1,000. At the present time this technology stands alone in its capability to produce nanoparticles without using electrochemical procedures and to boost zeolite potential to a level never previously attained in the domain of living things.

During the TMA activation process, the electrons whose chemical links have been shattered by collisions revert to a distribution described as semiavailable—that is, they can be freed on the demand of the environment, particularly when it comes in contact with free radicals (those molecules having an electron missing, which is replaced from proteins constituting the membrane or nucleus of cells). Free radicals cause destructive chain reactions leading to all sorts of diseases. Their neutralization is obtained either directly, using substances carrying the missing electron, or by stimulation of the body's natural antiradical defenses.

It was an experiment on a pig farm that first attracted attention to the properties of TMAZ. This new zeolite had been spread over the ground to measure its capacity to neutralize odors, but the pigs were found to be eating it and seemingly as a result, they were no longer victims of infarction or the acute respiratory sicknesses that are common to farm-raised pigs. Lelas was intrigued by these results and experimented with the consumption of this mineral powder among his friends and colleagues. Interestingly, a strongly positive reaction was noticed in the course of a few months in relation to several health problems. And so in 1997 the first research was performed at Zagreb University Medical School and then at the Ruder Boscovic Institute (specializing in molecular medicine research). The project then spread to other research institutes, universities, clinics, and hospitals in Austria and later to Germany and the United States. Toxicological analyses in vitro and in vivo that were conducted parallel to these studies established the safety of TMAZ.

The public very quickly became interested in the positive effects noted in volunteers who had begun to use TMAZ as well as in those who had been using TMAZ for a longer period of time (friends, relatives and colleagues of the inventors). Doctors soon proposed its use to support and reinforce the medical treatment of a variety of conditions.

Clinical studies involved patients with cancer, diabetes, and liver or cardiovascular disease. Results of these investigations showed improvement when TMAZ was used in conjunction with medical treatment and during convalescence. Often its use was directly followed by a dramatic improvement in general health due to recovery of the body's immune system and natural antiradical defenses. Symptoms such as tiredness and pain decreased in intensity over a few days.

Basing his suggestion on the well-known antifungal and antibiotic qualities of zeolites, Lelas proposed testing TMAZ in dermatological conditions and on postsurgical skin lesions and ulcerations. In both instances healing was affected positively.

According to laboratory studies, TMAZ acts as a superantigen capable of significantly stimulating and reinforcing the chain reaction of immune regulation—that is, immunostimulation of natural defenses or immunosuppression, in the case of an uncontrolled immune response, or allergies.

Regarding lycopenomin, which is composed of tribomechanically activated zeolites (TMAZs), or clinoptilolites, we know that different products from the megamine-lycopenomin family have been enhanced by combining TMAZ with dolomite earth, nettle leaves, pollen, and propolis. In tests of lycopenomin subjects were also given selenium, lycopene, and vitamin C. This resulted in the development of food supplements with an exceptional antioxidant capacity, which increases an organism's natural defenses.

Microparticles of zeolite could provide a major advance in the areas of illness prevention and sports medicine and can positively effect general tiredness. The importance of using antioxidant supplements in addition to prescribed medicines is generally recognized for many sicknesses in which oxidizing stress is high, in particular for instances of diabetes and cancer. The use of lycopenomin, which has no undesirable side effects, plays an important part in current research on anti-ageing substances by reinforcing vitality and slowing down organic ageing resulting from the constant and insidious action of free radicals. Zeolite microparticles are thus at the meeting point between natural and classical, or allopathic, approaches to health. This innovative food supplement does indeed interest high-level medical and scientific researchers and has received a recommendation from the European Academy of Interdisciplinary Medicine for its regulatory action on cell metabolism.

But the benefits of zeolites are not newly discovered. Tribomechanically activated zeolite and the procedure that produces it have been used experimentally for more than ten years in solving various problems in agricultural production. Certain minerals such as calcite, dolomite, and other calcium and magnesium carbonates that have been micronized through tribomechanical activation have been very effective protecting plants from various parasites. Calcite, either alone or mixed with manure, has been shown to be a good fertilizer that shortens required growing time and improves both the quantity and quality of the yield. And calcite mixed with manure significantly lessens the unpleasant odor of composting material when mixed with organic waste and accelerates the composting process.

TMAZ has also been used successfully in the production of cosmetics. Its direct application in powder form soothes nettle rash, allergic reactions, scars, scabs, wounds, and burns and when applied before washing hair or when mixed with shampoo, it eliminates dandruff. It can also be used as a skin peel, either dry or mixed with creams. Finally, it has been shown to help eliminate wrinkles when applied dry or mixed with a moisturizer.

In the past few years TMAZ has also proved effective in the treatment of various human and animal diseases.

1. Cancer. It has proved to aid in fighting cancer of the skin, cervix, breast, ovaries, prostate, liver or spleen, small or large intestine, lungs, bone, stomach, bladder, tongue, and thyroid.[2]

TMAZ has undergone tests with a variety of patients suffering from a range of malignancies and diseases—cancer of the protate, liver, intestines, cervix, pancreas, and lungs (some metastasized) and Crohn's disease—an in all subjects overall condition improved after taking TMAZ in capsule form. Positive results included weight gain, disappearance of some symptoms, and improved mobility.

How exactly do zeolites work to improve the condition of such patients? They possess size and shape selectivity and the possibility of metallo-enzyme mimicry and immuno-modulatory activity. As such, accumulating evidence has indicated that zeolites play an important role in regulation of the immune system. It has been reported that silica, silicates, and aluminosilicates act as nonspecific immuno-stimulators, similarly to superantigens.[3] Superantigens, a class of immuno-stimulatory and disease-causing proteins of bacterial and viral origin, have the ability to activate a relatively large fraction (5 percent to 20 percent) of our T-cell population.

Previous results have shown that clinoptilolite treatment of mice and dogs suffering various tumor types have led to improvement of their overall health, prolonged lifespan, and decrease in tumor size.[4] In addition, toxicological studies on mice and rats have demonstrated that clinoptilolite treatment has no negative effect.[5]

2. The circulatory system. TMAZ has also contributed to the stabilization and optimization of the functioning of the circulatory system and to improvement in blood pressure; reduction of the size of varicose veins; and reduction of and recovery from edema, swollen veins, hemorrhoids, and enlarged capillaries.

TMAZ has also aided in strengthening the heart muscle and accelerating post-heart attack recuperation and in improving the levels of cholesterol, triglycerides, and hemoglobin in the blood.

3. Digestive system. Zeolites have been shown to aid in the stabilization and optimal regulation of the digestive system, including the elimination of and recuperation from heartburn and stomach and duodenal ulcers.

4. Rheumatic disorders. TMAZ acts to help treat all types of rheumatic disorders, including sciatica, discopathy, spondilosis, arthritis, and rheumatic arthritis.

5. Kidney function. TMAZ produces a diuretic effect, improves kidney function, and aids in the treatment of kidney infections.

6. Skin diseases and wounds; skin quality. TMAZ is useful in the treatment of seborrhea, dermatitis, herpes (all types), psoriasis, and other skin ailments, through either peroral intake or its application in powder form. Direct application also helps in healing and pain relief of wounds and minor burns and in the quick and complete elimination of various fungal infections of the skin and mucous membrane. Overall, TMAZ can increase skin's moisture and resistance to negative external factors such as UV rays.

7. Diabetes Mellitus. After use of TMAZ, most of those tested showed a clear stabilization or decrease in the level of sugar in the blood.

8. Endocrine Glands. TMAZ optimizes endocrine gland activity, especially that of the lymph nodes.

9. Periodontosis. TMAZ aides in the treatment of periodontosis and the elimination of microorganisms in the mouth when applied directly to the gums or added to toothpaste.

10. Neuro-psychiatric effects. TMAZ improves overall disposition; successfully treats insomnia, neurosis, and depression; and assists in the treatment of epilepsy, schizophrenia, Alzheimer's disease, and Parkinson's disease.

11. Increasing Endurance. Zeolites contribute to overall increased endurance in situations of great physical effort and to the reduction or elimination of pain resulting from such activity.

Appendix 4
RESOURCES

American Longevity

1-888-441-4184

www.american-longevity.com

This Web site offers links to a variety of colloidal products as well as links to information from Dr. Joel Wallach on colloidal minerals.

CreoMed Inc.

4840 Sycamore Drive

Naples, Florida 34119

E-mail: information@creomed.com

www.creomed.com

This company is the U.S. source for Lycopenomin Active.®

The Grain and Salt Society

273 Fairway Drive

Asheville, NC 28805

1-800-TOP-SALT (867-7258)

www.celtic-seasalt.com

Quinton's Marine Plasma (sold under the trade name Marine Matrix in the United States) and other mineral-rich seawater products can be purchased from this source.

Lumière de Sel/Hasur Corporation
21 Industry Street, Unit 6
Aurora, Ontario
L4G 1X6 Canada
1-905-713-6300
Toll-free: 1-888-SEL-SALT (735-7258)
Fax: 1-905-713-6308
E-mail: info@lumieredesel.com or info@hasurcorporation.com
www.lumieredesel.com
This company is the source for both Himalayan salt and TMAZs.

Majestic Earth Minerals
www.majesticearth-minerals.com
This site is both a U.S. and international source for colloidal products specifically endorsed by Dr. Joel Wallach.

T. J. Clark, Inc.
1145 North 1100 West
St. George, UT 84770
1-800-228-0872
outside the United States: 1-435-634-0309
www.tjclarkinc.com
All-natural colloidal spring water can be purchased from this source.

NOTES

Chapter 1 A Brief History

1. *Lettres sur la chimie,* Justus Liebig (Paris: Éditions Baillière, 1845).
2. *Kreislauf des Lebens* (The Circulation of Life), Jacob Moleschott (Paris: Éditions Baillière, 1866).
3. Guillaume-Henri Schüssler, *Abrégé de thérapeutique biochimique* (Philadelphia: Boericke and Tafel, 1898).
4. Ibid.
5. Ibid.
6. L. Kolisko, *Sternenwirken in Erdstoffen* (Dornach, 1932).
7. Georges Faure, *Les métaux pour votre santé* (Saint Jean de Braye: Éditions Dangles, 1981).
8. Lernout and Tétau, *Comment soigner par les sels de Schüssler et par les minerals diluées et dynamisés* (Paris: Éditions Maloine, 1978).

Chapter 2 A Healthy Diet Is the Essential Foundation of Overall Good Health

1. Ann Wigmore, *The Wheatgrass Book* (Hippocrates Health Institute, 1985).
2. Anne Laroche-Walter, *Lait de vache, blancheur trompeuse* (Saint Julien en Genevois: Éditions Jouvence, 1998).
3. Hamaker and Weaver, *Survival of Civilization* (Burlingame, Calif.: Hamaker and Weaver Publishing, 1982).
4. See also Marie-France Muller, *Le chlorure de magnesium: un remède miracle inconnu* [Magnesium Chloride: An Ignored Miracle Remedy] (Saint Julien en Genevois: Éditions Jouvence, 1988).
5. Pierre Delbet, *Politique preventive du cancer* (Paris: Éditions Donoël, 1944).
6. Ibid.

Chapter 3 The Importance of Soil Quality

1. Tonita d'Raye, *Colloidal Minerals, Sparks of Life*, (Kletzer, Ore.: The Ten Minute Read Company, 1997), 6.

Chapter 4 Pollution: The Heavy Tribute Exacted by Modern Life

1. Americo Mosca, *Atoms in Agriculture* (Acres, 1974).
2. Sigmund Schmidt, *Can We Protect Our Bodies from the Poisons in the Surrounding Environment?* (Heidelberg, Germany: The German Research Center against Cancer).

Chapter 5 We Should All Live for 120 to 140 Years

1. From Joel D. Wallach, *Dead Doctors Don't Lie: Learn Why the Average Life Span of an M.D. Is only 58 Years!* (Wellness Publications, 1999).
2. Ibid.
3. Ibid.
4. Ibid.
5. Ibid.

Chapter 6 Supporting Research

1. From Joel D. Wallach, *Dead Doctors Don't Lie: Learn Why the Average Life Span of an M.D. Is only 58 Years!* (Wellness Publications, 1999).
2. Ibid.
3. Phyllis A. Balch and James Balch, *Prescription for Nutritional Healing: The A to Z Guide to Supplements* (New York: Avery Publishing Group, 2002).
4. G. Boden, X. Chen, J. Ruiz, et al. "Effects of vanadyl sulfate on carbohydrate and lipid metabolism in patients with non-insulin-dependent diabetes mellitus." *Metab Clin Exp* 45, no. 9 (1996): 1130–35.
5. Cited in *The Complete Guide to Your Emotions and Your Health*, Emrika Padus (Emmaus, Penn: Rodale Press, 1986).

Chapter 8 Earth, Soils, and Minerals

1. Dr. Jean-Pierre Willem, *Adieu vieillesse* (Paris: Édition du Dauphin, 2001).
2. For more information on the properties of clays and their therapeutic indications, see my book *L'argile pratique* (Saint Julien en Genevois: Édition Jouvence, 1998).
3. Ibid.
4. Claude Aubert, *L'agriculture biologique*, (Paris: Le Courrier du Livre, 1977).
5. Ibid.
6. Ibid.
7. See H. C. Geffroy, *Culture sans labours ni engrais* (La Vie Claire, 1981).

Chapter 9 Water: the Source of Life

1. André Simoneton, *Radiations des aliments, ondes humaines et santé* (Paris: Le Courrier du Livre, 1977).
2. Ibid.
3. Ibid.

Chapter 10 The Body: A Compound of Minerals and Trace Elements

1. See also Christopher Vasey, *The Acid–Alkaline Diet for Optimum Health* (Rochester, Vt: Inner Traditions, 2003).

Chapter 12 Colloidal Minerals: Sparks of Life

1. Tonita d'Raye, *Colloidal Minerals, Sparks of Life* (Kletzer, Ore.: The Ten Minute Read Company, 1997), 8.
2. From U.S. Senate Document 264, 74th Congress, Second Session, 1936.
3. Frederic Macy, "Chemistry's Miraculous Colloids," *Reader's Digest*, March 1936.
4. The story of Macy's demonstration was published in the March 1936 issue of *Reader's Digest*.

Chapter 13 The Role of Trace Elements

1. From Dr. Wessberge's 1918 doctoral thesis presented at the Sorbonne.
2. Lily Kolisko, *Physiologischer und physikalischer Nachweis der Wirkung kleinster Entitäten* (Stuttgart: Arbeitsgemeinschaft anthroposophischer Aerzte).
3. See Victor Bott, *Spiritual Science and the Art of Healing: Rudolf Steiner's Anthroposophical Medicine* (Rochester, Vt.: Healing Arts Press, 1996).
4. *Le vrai problème des oligo-éléments,* Center for the Research and Application of Trace Elements.
5. *La médecine biodynamique* (Paris: Éditions Jollois, 1999).
6. Paris: Librairie Maloine, 1979.

Chapter 14 Two Natural Sources of Colloidal Mineral Complexes

1. J. P. Willem, *Adieu vieillesse* [Good Bye to Old Age] (Paris: Éditions du Dauphin, 2001).
2. To learn more, see Fritz-Albert Popp, *La biologie de la lumière* [Light Biology] (Belgium: Éditions Marco Pietteur).
3. Andre Passebecq and Jean-Marc Soulier, *Plasma humain et plasma marin: etude comparée des propriétés thérapeutiques des preparations d'eau de mer* (Paris: Éditions Nouvelles Presses Internationales, 1991).

4. Bensch, "Vertus thérapeutiques de l'eau de mer" [Therapeutic properties of Seawater], *Journal du Médecin* (1966).

5. Michel Dogna, *Verités-Santé Pratique* (October 23, 1999).

Appendix 2: Himalayan Crystal Salt

1. Barbara Hendel and Peter Ferreira, *Wasser und Salz, Urquell des Lebens* (Köln, Germany: Ina Verlag, 2001).

Appendix 3: Tribomechanically Activated Zeolites (TMAZs)

1. M. Colic and K. Pavelic, "Molecular mechanisms of anticancer activity of natural dietetic products" *Journal of Molecular Medicine* (July 12, 2000).

2. K. Pavelic, M. Hadzija, et. al., "Natural zeolite clinoptilolite: new adjuvant in anticancer therapy," *Journal of Molecular Medicine* (January 2001).

3. (n.a.), "Immuno-stimulatory effect of natural clinoptilolite as a possible mechanism of antimetastatic ability," *Journal of Cancer Research and Clinical Oncology* (September 2001).

4. I. Martin-Kleiner, Z. Flegar-Mestric, et. al., "The effects of the zeolite clinoptilolite on serum chemistry and hematopoiesis in mice," *Food and Chemical Toxicology*, vol. 39 (2001): 717–27.

5. Ibid.

BIBLIOGRAPHY

Barefoot, Robert R., and Carl M. Reich. *The Calcium Factor: The Scientific Secret of Health and Youth.* Wickenburg: Bokar Consultants, 2002.

Bergson, Louis. *Creative Evolution.* Greenwood Press, 1975.

Bott, Victor. *Spiritual Science and the Art of Healing: Rudolf Steiner's Anthroposophical Medicine.* Rochester, Vt.: Inner Traditions, 1996.

Crow, W. B. *Precious Stones: Their Occult Powers.* Yorkville, Maine: RedWheel/Weiser, 1980.

D'Raye, Tonita. *Colloidal Minerals, Sparks of Life.* The Ten Minute Read Company, 1997.

Hamaker, John D., and Donald Weaver. *Survival of Civilization.* Seymour, Mo.: Hamaker and Weaver, 1982.

Liebig, Justus. *Familiar Letters of Chemistry in its Relation to Physiology, Dietetics, Agriculture, Commerce, and Political Economy.* Continuum Publishing Group, 2004.

Lovelock, James. *The Ages of Gaia.* New York: Bantam, 1990.

———. *Gaia: A New Look at Life on Earth.* Oxford: Oxford University Press, 1986.

Mosca, Americo. *Atoms in Agriculture.* Acres, 1974.

Padus, Emrika. *The Complete Guide to Your Emotions and Health.* Emmaus, Pa.: Rodale Press, 1990.

Vasey, Christopher. *The Acid–Alkaline Diet for Optimum Health.* Rochester, Vt.: Healing Arts Press, 2003.

Wallach, Joel. *Dead Doctors Don't Lie: Learn Why the Average Life Span of an M.D. Is Only 58 Years!* Wellness Publications, 1999.

Wigmore, Ann. *The Wheatgrass Book.* New York: Avery Publishing Group, 1984.

INDEX

BOOKS OF RELATED INTEREST

The Acid–Alkaline Diet for Optimum Health
Restore Your Health by Creating Balance in Your Diet
by Christopher Vasey, N.D.

Nutrition and Mental Illness
An Orthomolecular Approach to Balancing Body Chemistry
by Carl C. Pfeiffer, Ph.D., M.D.

The High Blood Pressure Solution
A Scientifically Proven Program for Preventing
Strokes and Heart Disease
by Richard D. Moore, M.D., Ph.D.

Prickly Pear Cactus Medicine
Treatments for Diabetes, Cholesterol, and the Immune System
by Ran Knishinsky

The Clay Cure
Natural Healing from the Earth
by Ran Knishinsky

The Whole Food Bible
How to Select & Prepare Safe, Healthful Foods
by Chris Kilham

Genetically Engineered Food: Changing the Nature of Nature
What You Need to Know to Protect Yourself,
Your Family, and Our Planet
by Martin Teitel, Ph.D., and Kimberly A. Wilson

Medical Herbalism
The Science and Practice of Herbal Medicine
by David Hoffmann, F.N.I.M.H.

Inner Traditions • Bear & Company
P.O. Box 388
Rochester, VT 05767
1-800-246-8648
www.InnerTraditions.com

Or contact your local bookseller